EIGHT QUESTIONS
YOU SHOULD ASK ABOUT OUR
HEALTH CARE SYSTEM

(EVEN IF THE ANSWERS MAKE YOU SICK)

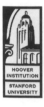

The Hoover Institution gratefully acknowledges
the following individuals and foundations
for their significant support of the
Working Group on Health Care Policy
and this publication:

LYNDE AND HARRY BRADLEY FOUNDATION

EIGHT QUESTIONS YOU SHOULD ASK ABOUT OUR HEALTH CARE SYSTEM

(EVEN IF THE ANSWERS MAKE YOU SICK)

Charles E. Phelps

HOOVER INSTITUTION PRESS
Stanford University | Stanford, California

The Hoover Institution on War, Revolution and Peace, founded at Stanford University in 1919 by Herbert Hoover, who went on to become the thirty-first president of the United States, is an interdisciplinary research center for advanced study on domestic and international affairs. The views expressed in its publications are entirely those of the authors and do not necessarily reflect the views of the staff, officers, or Board of Overseers of the Hoover Institution.

www.hoover.org

Hoover Institution Press Publication No. 581

Hoover Institution at Leland Stanford Junior University,
Stanford, California, 94305–6010

First printing 2010

16 15 14 13 12 11 10   9 8 7 6 5 4 3 2 1

Manufactured in the United States of America

Illustration on page 106 by Taylor Jones.

Hoover Institution Press has no responsibility for the persistence or accuracy of URLs for external or third-party internet websites referred to in this publication, and does not guarantee that any content on such websites is, or will remain, accurate or appropriate.

The paper used in this publication meets the minimum Requirements of the American National Standard for Information Sciences—Permanence of Paper for Printed Library Materials, ANSI/NISO Z39.48–1992. ⊗

Cataloging-in-Publication Data is available from the Library of Congress
ISBN-13: 978-0-8179-1054-9 (cloth. : alk. paper)
ISBN-13: 978-0-8179-1056-3 (e-book)

To Dale—our time has just begun, once again.

CONTENTS

Contents

FOREWORD

Remarkable advances in health care have occurred during the past sixty years. Dramatic improvements in diagnostic and therapeutic strategies, as well as significant advances in medical technologies, pharmaceuticals, and surgical procedures have extended the length of life and greatly improved its quality as well. For example, progress in the treatment of cardiovascular disease has reduced, by more than a 50 percent, the U.S. death rate from heart attacks accounting for nearly all the increases in the expected life-span in the United States since 1950.

Despite such extraordinary progress, however, U.S. health care faces serious challenges. The problem is not so much that health care spending is high, but that a significant portion of that spending fails to provide good value. As spending grows, an increasing number of people are unable to afford health insurance. The fiscal burden of federal and state health care entitlement programs, such as Medicare and Medicaid, can no longer be sustained without either deep reductions in other public programs or sharply higher taxes. Diverting both public and private resources from more productive uses has become a serious problem.

The debate over the direction of U.S. health care policy is occupying center stage in the domestic policy arena now and will so during the coming years. The promise of future medical advances stemming from the mapping of the human genome, nanotechnology, and other innovations is bright. But progress will require us to transcend the terms of the current debate, which are often expressed as the competing goals of universal insurance and cost control. The fundamental challenge is to devise public policies that enable more Americans to get better value for their health care dollar and foster appropriate innovations that extend and improve life. Key principles that guide policy formation should include the central role of individual choice and competitive markets in financing and delivering health services, individual responsibility for health behaviors and decisions, and appropriate guidelines for government intervention in health care markets.

The current core membership of the Hoover Institution's Working Group on Health Care Policy includes Scott W. Atlas, John F. Cogan, R. Glenn Hubbard, Daniel P. Kessler, Mark V. Pauly, and Charles E. Phelps.

JOHN RAISIAN
Tad and Diane Taube Director,
Hoover Institution, Stanford University
Stanford, California

PREFACE

First, a couple of things that this book does *not* do. It does not comment specifically on current legislation, still under debate in the House and Senate as this book goes to press in early 2010, except for noting sins of commission and omission in the final chapter. In addition, the book focuses entirely on the U.S. health care system, albeit with some comparisons to other nations to put our data into context.

Second, this book does not offer my own recommendations (and the logic underlying them) for a proper fix for the system. I suspect that the reader can tease out my preferences, which would include elimination of the tax subsidy for employer-paid insurance, an emphasis on high-deductible plans such as Health Savings Accounts (HSAs), and a massive effort to deal with the problems of obesity, tobacco, and alcohol abuse.

What do I intend to accomplish with this book? I hope it will help intelligent and interested citizens to become more informed about important economic issues that are central to fixing our health care system. I also hope it will be accessible to those without formal economic training, while at the same time aiding and provoking serious discussion about these issues.

Charles E. Phelps
Gualala, California
March 2010

ACKNOWLEDGMENTS

I extend my appreciation to the Hoover Institution at Stanford University for making this book possible. I particularly thank John Cogan for the lead role he played in this endeavor; Dan Kessler for very helpful comments on a draft; and John Raisian for his assistance in making it happen.

I have also received valuable comments on an earlier draft from many friends whom I wish to acknowledge, especially Bruce Bueno de Mesquita (NYU and Hoover Institution), Debbie Freund (Syracuse University), Victor Fuchs (Stanford), Tom Jackson (University of Rochester), Andy Markovits (University of Michigan), and my brothers, Hugh Phelps, M.D., and especially Lew Phelps.

CHAPTER **1**

How Did We Get into This Mess, and Why Will It Get Worse?

A t the writing of this book, Congress grapples to re-form the U.S. health care system. Whatever it enacts will merely stand as the beginning of a long endeavor to change and control health care spending in the United States. History tells us as much: when Congress enacted Medicare and Medicaid in 1965, nobody understood the consequences, and subsequent legislation has massively changed the structure and purposes of both. During the same period, other large federal governmental health care systems also changed markedly, most notably health care and insurance for military personnel, retirees, and their families. We can expect nothing different from any nationwide reforms affecting the entire health care system.

In order to understand the likely consequences of federal legislation and the private sector response, it is useful to understand how the current system evolved and

1

then to dig into some of the details about how the health care sector behaves. Subsequent chapters delve into some of these issues with a new slant: Eight Questions You Should Ask About Our Health Care System (Even if the Answers Make You Sick). Some of them have scary implications, but you *do* need to ask.

A quick overview

The U.S. health care sector is an amazing endeavor. It produces about one-sixth of the nation's Gross Domestic Product (GDP). If viewed as a separate country, it would rank as the seventh largest economy in the world, not far behind the United Kingdom and France and just ahead of Italy. It has not always been this way. Half a century ago, the United States and Canada spent about 6 percent of their GDPs on health care. Health spending in the United States has increased faster than that of other nations, and our 16 percent GDP share exceeds that of any other nation by a considerable amount.

Some of this comes as no surprise to those who have studied the U.S. health care system over the years. Figure 1.1 shows a remarkably strong pattern between per capita income and medical spending. It's easy to see that per capita income goes a long way toward explaining why the United States spends so much on health care: we are wealthier than any other nation, and wealth leads to more spending on health care in a very systematic fash-

FIGURE 1.1
National Income and Medical Spending
(US Dollars, 2006)

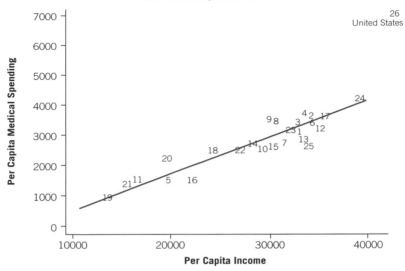

Per Capita Income

Legend for Figures 1.1 through 1.4		
1. Australia	10. Greece	19. Poland
2. Austria	11. Hungary	20. Portugal
3. Belgium	12. Iceland	21. Slovak Republic
4. Canada	13. Ireland	22. Spain
5. Czech Republic	14. Italy	23. Sweden
6. Denmark	15. Japan	24. Switzerland
7. Finland	16. South Korea	25. United Kingdom
8. France	17. Netherlands	26. United States
9. Germany	18. New Zealand	

Data source: OECD

ion. But the United States sits far above the trend line drawn through the other countries in this graph.

One of the remarkable things about the data portrayed in Figure 1.1 is that the organization of the health care

3

financing and delivery systems of the nations shown has almost nothing to do with per capita spending. Very close to the trend line, we find nations such as Canada (social insurance, private production of health care), Germany and Japan (mixed sources of insurance, private production of health care), Great Britain (social insurance and health care through the British National Health Service), and Sweden (county-level financing and control of health care). None of this seems to matter: per capita income tells almost the entire story, except for the United States.

That the United States sits far above the trend line suggests that something else affects our health care spending. One difference is compensation of our health care providers. Doctors in the United States have incomes significantly higher (relative to the average worker's income) than doctors in most other nations. We have a relatively decentralized financing system with no central budget constraints. We also invest more in technology. And we have different health habits. All of these things contribute to the United States' position above the trend line in Figure 1.1.

Despite common political rhetoric that "health care is a necessity" or "health care is a right," these data contain another surprise to many: health care acts much more like a luxury than a necessity. In standard economics jargon, spending on a necessity grows less rapidly than income growth, and spending on luxury goods grows faster than income growth. In these data, medical spending grows about 25 percent faster than the rate of income growth.

This graph contains a lesson for the future as well: as our per capita income grows in the future, so will our medical spending. Since we can expect income growth in the future (despite the recession of 2008–2009), we can expect growth in both the level of spending and the GDP share. It will inexorably grow no matter what governmental policies emerge or what reforms Congress might enact or modify through the years. Figure 1.1 tells us that.

Figures 1.2 and 1.3 show something even more disquieting. Despite outspending the rest of the world for medical care, our health outcomes are depressingly low. Whether measured by life expectancy at birth (Figure 1.2) or the more-responsive infant death rate (Figure 1.3), it is easy to see that we are not getting as much bang for the buck as other nations do. (As in Figure 1.1, the trend lines here go through the other countries in the graphs.) Many nations, in fact, have much lower infant mortality and higher life expectancy than the United States, often while spending about half as much per person as we do. This discrepancy between spending and outcomes drives much of the concern about our health care system.

One might ask if the life expectancy data in Figure 1.2 don't just reflect the infant mortality rates in Figure 1.3, but with pretty much the same outcomes in every country for those who survive birth. The answer again is a very disquieting "no." Figure 1.4 shows the graph of life

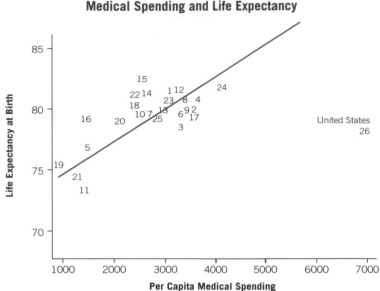

FIGURE 1.2
Medical Spending and Life Expectancy

Note: For a key explaining what number represents which nation in this figure, please refer back to the legend that appears with Figure 1.1 on page 3.
Data source: OECD

expectancy at age twenty-five for the same countries graphed against medical spending per capita.[1] The United States still looms as a larger outlier. Country number fifteen, Japan, again gets the best outcome for about half of our per capita spending. The predicted value for the United States using a line fitting the other twenty-five

---

1. The story looks almost exactly the same if one looks at life expectancy at age fifty or almost any other age, once the effects of infant mortality are eliminated.

6

FIGURE 1.3
Medical Spending and Infant Mortality

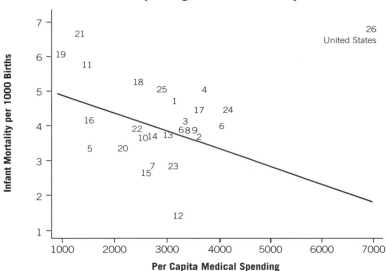

Note: For a key explaining what number represents which nation in this figure, please refer back to the legend that appears with Figure 1.1 on page 3.
Data source: OECD

nations in this graph is ninety-two years of life expectancy (given our medical spending rates), versus the actual outcome of just under eighty-four years. Those eight years of missing life expectancy do not come from the higher infant mortality rates we have; they come from something else.

Nobody can rightfully claim to understand fully why we get such relatively poor results for our medical spending efforts. Many things contribute to our high spending and poor outcomes. The United States has a greater de-

7

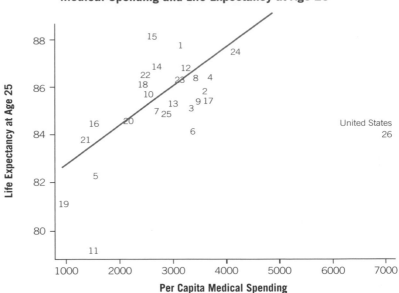

FIGURE 1.4
Medical Spending and Life Expectancy at Age 25

Note: For a key explaining what number represents which nation in this figure, please refer back to the legend that appears with Figure 1.1 on page 3.
Data source: www.worldlifeexpectancy.com

gree of population heterogeneity than do most other nations.[2] Our lifestyle habits are better on some dimensions than other nations' (most notably regarding tobacco use)

---

2. This can affect health outcomes in many ways. For example, if the patient is not fluent in English and the doctor and nurse speak only English, things won't work as well as if they could communicate perfectly. Many other issues arise with heterogeneity, including genetic differences and lifestyle differences, which can affect health outcomes as we commonly measure them.

TABLE 1.1
Health Care Spending in the US—A Half-Century of Change
(Billions of dollars)

Year	Actual Dollars	Inflation Adjusted (2005 $)	Constant Population 2005	Medical Price Adjustment	Constant Age Mix
1960	23	153	255	672	769
1970	63	316	461	961	
1980	215	510	668	1260	
1990	608	908	1082	1483	
2000	1140	1293	1362	1514	
2010	2600	2292	2233	2012	2012
Ratio of 2010/1960	113	15	8.8	3.0	2.6

Data source: Health United States, 2009, US Department of Health and Human Services, National Center for Health Statistics, Hyattsville, MD, 2010, Table 123.

but worse on others (most notably obesity). Subsequent chapters in this book detail the importance of these lifestyle issues. All we need to know at this point comes directly out of Figures 1.1 through 1.4: we spend much more per person than do other nations (much, but not all, of that difference arising because of our income level) and we don't have health outcomes as good as many other nations, all of whom we outspend.

Examining the spending changes: The overall change in dollars spent on health care over the past half century is mind-numbing. Table 1.1 shows the relevant data in decade-wide intervals from 1960 to 2010 (with a bit of extrapolation to the final numbers). A useful way to understand these changes parses out the shifts through time. Begin with the real mind-boggler: we have grown from $23 billion in 1960 to approximately $2.6 trillion by the end of 2010, the latter number 113 times larger than the former. How on earth did we get more than a hundred-fold increase in medical spending over a fifty-year period?

The second column of table 1.1 tells much of the story: it's simple inflation. If we adjust the data in column one so that everything appears in constant 2005 dollars, the earlier numbers rise (to adjust for inflation) so that the ratio of 2010 to 1960 spending is 15. A further adjustment assumes that the population was the same in 1960 as in 2010, hence taking out the effect of population growth in the numbers.[3] The ratio now falls to 8.8, representing an annual compound growth rate of 4.4 percent.

The next column takes a potentially risky step: it adjusts for the change in the relative prices of medical care versus all other goods and services. If the Consumer Price Index (CPI) adjustment did this just right, this would adjust for changes in the relative payments to providers of health care (hospitals, doctors, etc.) for services with constant quality. But of course quality has changed immensely over that half century, and only some of those changes get captured in the CPI relative price adjust-

---

3. This does the same thing as looking at "per capita spending" rates would do, except that these are total spending in billions of dollars instead of per capita spending rates.

ment. So some of the 8.8 factor is pricing of services and some of it is increases in quality. We have no really good way to tell how much of the 8.8 factor is quality change. What we do know is that after the relative price adjustment, we still see an increase by a factor of about 3.0 in medical spending in the past half century, even after making all of these adjustments. Adjusting finally for the shift in age mix (older people use more health care), we still have a 2.6 multiplier.

What does the 2.6 factor represent? Many observers (myself included) attribute this to changes in technology. The world of health care is vastly different now than it was in 1960. We have seen incredible changes in imaging tools for diagnosis, far-less-invasive surgery, new pharmaceutical treatments for physical and mental illnesses, and many other changes (a few of which Chapter Three goes over in more detail).

The point can be made simply: If you had your choice of 1960s medicine at 1960s prices or 2010 medicine at 2010 prices, which would you choose? For many (myself definitely included), the choice is simple: 2010 dominates 1960.

The baby boom's echo: One more factor affects both the past history of medical spending and projections into the future. The baby boom following the end of World War II had many consequences for our economy in the subsequent decades, but none more important than the effects on health care costs, past and future. Figure 1.5 shows

FIGURE 1.5a

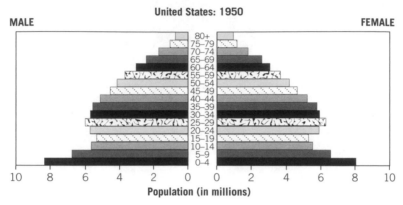

United States: 1950

Data source: US Census Bureau

the key data in what demographers call a population pyramid.

Reading these charts is easy and informative. The left side shows the number of males, the right side the number of females, and each "layer" shows a different age group, youngest at the bottom. Figure 1.5a shows the U.S. population in 1950. It looks like a classic population pyramid from age twenty upward. It is "thin-waisted" for the young age groups either with reduced birth rates (because many young potential fathers were overseas during World War II) or early deaths (of young soldiers). The bottom row of Figure 1.5a shows the beginning of the baby boom when the soldiers returned from the war and began to form families and father children.

Now fast-forward for fifty years to the 2000 population

12

FIGURE 1.5b

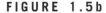

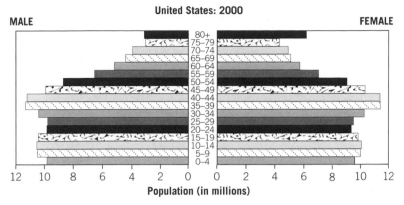

Data source: US Census Bureau

pyramid (Figure 1.5b). The pyramid (like many Americans) has a pretty nice set of "love handles" at its waist. That's the baby boomers in their forties. By 2025 (Figure 1.5c) they're aging into the Medicare set, and the pyramid has pretty much become a column. By 2050 (Figure 1.5d) the shape has completely changed, becoming very top-heavy.

The scary part of these population trends comes from the world of public finance. Members of the working-age population (those about twenty to sixty-five) support those layers below them (their children) and those above them (their parents and grandparents). The 1950 pyramid shows many workers to provide support for the non-workers. That still held in 2000, with the baby boomers in their prime productive years. By 2025, the ratio will

13

FIGURE 1.5c

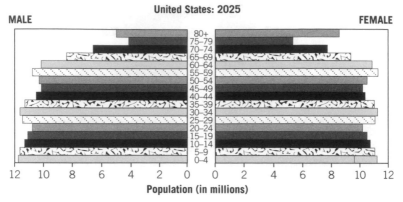

Data source: US Census Bureau

FIGURE 1.5d

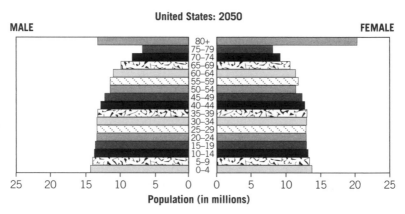

Data source: US Census Bureau

14

have shifted considerably, and the projections to 2050 show a very large fraction of the population as non-workers compared with the fraction of working age.

Our system of Social Security in the United States is not a retirement program in the sense that people save and invest their own money for use in retirement years. Rather, it is partly a "pay as you go" system, with Social Security taxes on current workers funding the retirement payments to those beyond age sixty-five.[4] The same is true of the Medicare Trust Fund, with the added wrinkle (if you'll pardon the expression) that as humans age, their use of medical care accelerates because their bodies wear out faster. The Social Security-like financing system works fine when the ratio of workers to non-workers is favorable, but it becomes more troublesome when the pyramid looks like the 2025 version, and is even more problematic in the 2050 version. The upper layer of the 2050 pyramid is particularly scary, since people over age eighty consume far more medical care than younger people do. Somehow the Medicare Trust Fund has to deal with these issues over time.

With these macro-economic issues out of the way (spending and population trends), let's look at health care as individuals know it. We'll look at things from the consumers' point of view, and then from the medical care suppliers' point of view.

---

4. There are complicated trust fund issues here. Current workers pay into the Social Security and Medicare Trust Funds at about the same rate that funds flow out of that same fund to retirees. The retirees' own contributions would not support the funds they currently receive.

Key issues on the consumers' side of the market

Health insurance changes the way we use health care:
Most (but not all) people in the United States have
health insurance of some sort to help pay for their medical costs. This insurance operates differently than other
types of insurance. If you bang up your car or your home
gets damaged, an appraiser (or several repair estimates)
provides the basis for the insurance payment. Using a
specific example, if the damage costs $2,000 to fix, the
insurance company pays you $2,000 less any amount of
deductible that the insurance plan you chose specifies
(say, $500). Thus, $2,000 in damages gets you a check
for $1,500. You can use it to fix the car or you can drive
around with the damaged car and spend the $1,500 on
food, a new refrigerator in your kitchen, a vacation week-
end at some golf resort, or a case of really, really nice
wine. But you don't have to fix your car to get the
money. It's just money.

With health insurance, things don't work that way.
Since there's no easy way for an appraiser to estimate the
damage to your body, health insurance invariably pays a
different way. It pays for medical care that you decide to
buy. Sometimes you pay, for example, a $20 copayment
for a doctor visit that would have cost $225 if you didn't
have insurance. Sometimes the insurance pays for 80
percent of the doctor's bill, and you pay the remaining
20 percent. But in every case, *it reduces the price you pay
when you make the decision about getting treated.* It's not

16

"just money," but rather it's "funny money." You only get something from your insurance when you buy medical care.

To economists, this is a key issue. Health insurance reduces the price you pay at the point of purchase. That's how health insurance reduces the financial risk that arises from illnesses and injuries. But we know that when people face lower prices for things, they buy more. This is true also in health care. Chapter Two presents the evidence on how much this matters, but for now, we just need to know two things: health insurance reduces prices that people pay at decision time; and this affects their choices.

Taken to the extreme, it's easy to see how this works. When we make choices between buying a lower-cost Chevy or a really snazzy BMW, we ask ourselves, "Does the extra cost of the BMW bring me enough extra pleasure to justify the extra cost?" If so, we drive a BMW. If not, we drive a Chevy. But in medical care, the insurance causes us to ask a different question: "Can this procedure provide me with any possible benefit above the risks and pain of doing it?" If so, we tell the doctor, "Sure, go ahead." If not, we say, "No thanks, I'd rather just wait it out." Even if the insurance does not cover the procedure fully, the same type of shift occurs in most of the decisions we make with our doctors, dentists, and other health care providers.

Our health insurance comes from many sources: For many people in the United States, the government provides health insurance coverage.[5] For those over sixty-five and some others, it's Medicare (about 36 million total). For many people in low-income families (about 42 million), it's Medicaid and the State Children's Health Insurance Program (SCHIP), both of which are state-federal partnerships with an income test. Active-duty and retired military personnel, reservists, and their families get coverage through TRICARE, and low-income veterans can receive care through the Department of Veterans Affairs. Through these and other programs, a bit over a quarter of the U.S. population currently has health care coverage from the government.[6]

The bulk of health insurance in the United States comes through the places people work. Employer-provided health insurance covers about 157 million people (workers and their families) and has been the cornerstone of the health care financing system for well over half a century. For most workers, part of this cost comes as a deduction from their paychecks, but most of the cost is hidden as an "employer contribution." As shown in Chapter Four, this employer-based financing contains numerous pitfalls, but is nevertheless a staple of the U.S. health care system. About 14 million people just go out

---

5. Data source: http://www.statehealthfacts.org (Kaiser Family Foundation).

6. The fraction of all health dollars (45 percent in 2006) that flows through government programs will soon surpass 50 percent even without any legislative changes because of the higher per-person spending for those in the Medicare program and the growing over-65 population.

and buy health insurance as they would buy auto or homeowners' insurance. This is relatively more costly than employer-paid insurance for a number of reasons (most notably the higher administrative costs of dealing with people one at a time rather than in large-group purchases), and it carries no tax break, as does employer-paid insurance, so most people choose the employer-provided option when available, even if it's not exactly the insurance coverage they might choose on their own.

Finally, a number of people go without health insurance. Members of this group—estimated at 46 million in 2009—pay for medical care out of pocket, or they go to hospital clinics and emergency rooms and hope that they won't be charged. On average, about 5 percent of the cost of operating a typical hospital in the United States is "bad debt and charity care," a combined total reflecting the fluidity between the categories.[7]

Key issues on the provider side

While later chapters will deal with specific issues relating to providers of health care services, drugs, and devices, this section sets out two specific ideas. First, I will show how the relative importance of various parts of the health

7. Put simply, the hospital will try to get you to pay; if you don't, it can either write it off as a bad debt after trying to collect from you or it can say, "OK, it was charity care." Since hospitals need to provide some charity care to justify their exemption from income taxes, it's not hard

TABLE 1.2
Market Shares by Sector

Year	Hospital	Physician	Pharma-Drugs	Nursing Homes	Other
1960	39	23	12	3	23
1970	44	22	9	6	19
1980	47	22	6	9	16
1990	41	26	7	9	17
2000	37	25	12	8	18
2010	37	25	14	7	17

Data source: Health United States, 2009, US Department of Health and Human Services, National Center for Health Statistics, Hyattsville, MD, 2010, Table 126.

care sector has shifted over the years, and briefly discuss some of the underlying forces creating these shifts. Second, I will discuss the types of organizations (and their presumed goals) in the various sectors.

Shifts in the locus of treatment: Table 1.2 shows the time pattern of the shares of the health care sector over the past half-century. The shares, by definition, add up to 100 percent in every year, but we must remember that the overall size of the economic pie has grown immensely during this period (see Table 1.1).

Two interesting trends appear in these data. First, hospital care increased in importance (market share) from 1960 to about 1980, peaking at 47 percent, and then fell

---

to understand why many bad debts eventually get classified as charity care.

steadily, settling in at about 37 percent now. The period of shrinkage came with the confluence of two completely different factors. First, new technology (arthroscopic and laparoscopic surgery) greatly reduced lengths of stay for patients receiving those interventions. Second, Medicare (followed shortly by most private insurance companies) changed the way it paid hospitals beginning in 1983, creating strong incentives to reduce length of stay for all patients. These factors combined to put the hospital budgets on a dramatically effective diet, and they shrank accordingly. In addition, part of this came from a shift to home health care, long-term care, and hospice care; some of these activities were directly linked with hospitals, while some were free-standing.

The other trend of note is pharmaceutical drugs. The cost share held by drugs fell steadily from 1960 to about 1980. The drug share actually halved during that period (from 12 percent of total medical spending to 6 percent), and then it grew rapidly (and continues to do so), now reaching 14 percent. Obviously, many new drugs came into the market during this period to treat heart disease, cancers, diabetes, mental illnesses, heartburn, and many other illnesses, not to mention the highly advertised lifestyle drugs such as those treating erectile dysfunction and male pattern baldness.

Another important change took place in 1980: the Bayh-Dole Act changed the way medical research could be patented. A subsequent section in this chapter describes this regulatory shift in more detail.

Diverse ownership patterns: The United States has a widely mixed set of institutional arrangements for providing various health care services. The form of ownership—for profit, not for profit, or governmental—can affect the goals, quality of care, and financial stability of the various health care service providers, so it's worth noting the way we deliver these services in our country.

Some nations, of course, mostly depend on governmental provision of health care, including (until recent political shifts) most socialist states (Soviet Union, People's Republic of China, and others), Great Britain, and Sweden. Others depend heavily on private provision of health care, including the United States, Canada, Germany, and Japan. Almost all of these latter nations have a mix of private and public provision of health care.

In the United States, the mix of private and public looks radically different depending on which part of the health care system you look at. For hospital care, about 70 percent of all hospital beds are in private *not-for-profit* hospitals, another 14 percent are private *for-profit* hospitals, and the remaining 16 percent are governmental hospitals (mostly county hospitals, either in large cities or in rural areas).

Nursing homes have participation from all three sectors as well, but the *for-profit* sector dominates with about three-quarters of the market, followed by 20 percent in the *not-for-profit* sector, and the remaining 5 percent provided in government facilities (mostly local governments).

22

Pharmaceutical production and sales are almost entirely for-profit in nature. The invention and manufacturing of pharmaceutical drugs is a worldwide industry, with major players located not only in the United States but in Switzerland, Italy, France, England, Germany, Japan, and many other developed nations. Retail sales (excluding those sold through the pharmacies of not-for-profit and governmental hospitals) are almost entirely on a for-profit basis, with a few national chains (CVS, Walmart, Rite Aid) dominating the market.

The government sector has a lock on only one area in the United States: public health. The public health system spans the domain of governance entities, beginning with myriad local departments of public health (usually county government), coordinated at the state level by corresponding state departments of health, which in turn interact with the U.S. Public Health Service. The most important branches of the Public Health Service are the Centers for Disease Control and Prevention (CDC), responsible for prevention and control of infectious and other diseases; the Centers for Medicare & Medicaid Services (CMS), which operates Medicare and coordinates with the fifty states, District of Columbia, and U.S. territories in their Medicaid programs; the National Institutes of Health (NIH), the major engine for biomedical research in the United States and worldwide; and the Food and Drug Administration (FDA), responsible for food safety and for regulation of drugs and medical devices entering the U.S. market (more about this issue follows in the next section). The U.S. Public Health Service, formed in 1798, is one of the oldest and most durable public agencies in our nation.

The legal context

Two branches of the law affect our health care system more than others: the tort (liability) system and the regulatory laws of the U.S. and state governments.

Medical malpractice law: The part of the legal system affecting health care delivery that has the highest visibility is our medical malpractice structure. Malpractice law falls into the general domain of "tort" law, wherein persons who believe that they have been harmed inappropriately by others may sue them for damages. The harmed person (the plaintiff) must initiate the claim, and is almost always represented in court by a lawyer specializing in tort law or even more specialized in malpractice law, sometimes to the point of specializing in harms coming from a specific drug or procedure. Each state has its own medical malpractice law, the rules for which define the standards of liability, limits on damages, the ways the plaintiff's attorney can share in malpractice awards, and other aspects of the legal system.

Many observers believe that our medical malpractice system (or sometimes, more pointedly, the relatively high number of plaintiffs' lawyers specializing in medical malpractice) is the cause of our large and rapidly growing medical budget. If so, it is difficult to prove. Malpractice insurance costs (and malpractice awards) constitute only a few percent of the overall cost of health care and, more importantly, have not grown notably (as a share of the total health care "pie") over time. In order for malpractice costs to represent the *cause* of growing health care costs, the malpractice insurance and award costs would necessarily have to grow over time.

There is, of course, an indirect link: defensive medicine. Many health care providers state that they carry out numerous diagnostic tests (and undertake various procedures) only because of the threat of a lawsuit if something goes awry with the patient and they haven't "done everything possible" to test for or treat the cause of the patient's ailment. If so, then growing technological capabilities of the health care system (e.g., CT scans and magnetic resonance imaging) could lead to increased defensive medical spending.

Regulation: The health care system is the most highly regulated part of the U.S. economy. The government determines who can practice various medical professions (medicine, nursing, therapies of various sorts, pharmacy, psychology, etc.) through state licensing laws. The government also regulates the safety and quality of institutional providers (hospitals, nursing homes, etc.) and sets the prices these providers can charge—at least through Medicare and Medicaid (and, during some eras, throughout the health care system). The government also controls when new providers can enter the market (through state and local "certificate of need" programs of various sorts) and what pharmaceutical products can enter the market, through the FDA's drug regulatory arm. Perhaps the U.S. commercial aviation industry is equally regulated for safety issues, but there are no comparable restrictions on pricing or entry into the market as we find in the health care setting.

The creation and distribution of pharmaceutical products ("drugs" hereafter) deserves special mention. Drug makers ("Big Pharma" to some) operate with two distinctly different regulatory regimes. First, their inventions (new drugs and devices) can receive patent protection under general U.S. and international patent laws. The U.S. Constitution (Article 1, Section 8) created the right for the government to issue patents (and control copyright) and of Congress to have exclusive control over the terms thereof. The goal (as stated in the Constitution) is ". . . to promote the progress of science and useful arts, by securing for limited times to authors and inventors the exclusive right to their respective writings and discoveries."

Current patent law provides for a period of protection of twenty years (up from seventeen after 1994 international treaty negotiations), but the period of effective patent protection for new drugs and medical devices is considerably less (about ten to twelve years) because clinical testing of the drug consumes many years at the beginning of the patent.

The patent holder has the right to determine exclusively the use of the patent, including monopoly production of the patented product, licensing of the rights to produce to others (or combinations thereof), or the ability to simply exclude others from producing using the patented technology. Thus, patents grant a specific form of property rights to the patent holders, with the requirement that the holder of the right also has responsibility for protecting that right (commonly, by civil lawsuit in the tort system for patent infringement).

Separately from U.S. patent law, drug makers must carry out an extensive set of tests to measure the safety and efficacy of their products. These rules are enforced by the FDA, and are generally perceived as the most rigorous of any worldwide. Independently of whether a drug has received patent protection, the FDA requires multiple states of research to demonstrate both the safety of the drug (understanding that some drugs such as chemotherapy for cancer are intrinsically dangerous) and its efficacy (proof that it works). The costs of these studies are staggering—recent estimates put the total economic cost to bring a drug to market at $800 million per drug in 2000 and near $1 billion per drug now (DiMasi et al. 2003) although some dispute those figures (Goonzer 2004; D.W. Light 2005; DiMasi, Hansen, and Grabowski 2005).

Much of the research on drugs gets carried out by the drug companies directly. Industry sources state, for example, that about one thousand compounds are evaluated for each one that reaches the market. But much of the basic research underlying that effort is funded by the National Institutes of Health. The NIH annually funds over $25 billion in sponsored research, most of it carried out in medical schools across the United States. Many medical schools have NIH grant use exceeding $250 million per year, a few exceeding $1 billion per year.

A major turning point in the world of sponsored research occurred in 1980 with the passage of the Bayh-Dole Act, which transformed the way universities carried out biomedical research. Up to that point, any invention arising from NIH-sponsored research was owned by the NIH. But the NIH had little incentive or interest in commercializing the results of that research. The Bayh-Dole Act shifted the ownership of patents onto the universities producing the research. With visions of endless streams of patent royalties dancing in their heads, universities created and expanded offices of technology patenting and licensing, since the universities could use any forthcoming royalties for "scientific research and education." Recent reports show that U.S. universities annually produce more than three thousand patents and receive over $1.25 billion in royalty revenues under the Bayh-Dole Act.

Wrap-up

Our governments always have had, and always will have, a large role to play in our health care system. Tax laws have shaped the health sector both through non-taxation of health insurance premiums and through designation of some health care providers as tax-exempt not-for-profit organizations. Direct federal investment in research (mostly via the NIH) has spurred enormous technical changes in the health sector. Federal and state programs subsidize the training of health workers. And, of course, federal, state, and local governments have a key role in public health, dating back to 1798 with the founding of the U.S. Public Health Service. But even some of these important governmental interventions—most notably the tax treatment of health insurance paid by employers—occurred almost by accident.

Incentives also play an important part in the ways we produce and use health care. For consumers, these incentives arise through tax law, the ways health insurance changes the cost of health care when we use it, and the incentives to maintain our good health. In short, prices matter—a lot, in some cases. For producers of health care, incentives also matter a lot, with numerous events showing that if we change the incentives facing providers, they change their behavior, often quite radically.

The remainder of this book examines our health insurance system, improved technology, incentives for providers and consumers, and how all these things distort the practice of medicine while contributing to high costs. Finally, I will describe the real causes of death and disease and how education can move individual Americans toward better choices that will improve everyone's lives while reducing health care costs. Your take-home messages are these:

- The good, the bad, and the ugly. Our health care system contains much of each.
- Incentives and information. These are the ways to turn the bad and the ugly into the good.
- We have met the enemy, and they are us. Many (indeed, most) of our health problems (and subsequent medical care costs) arise from our own health habits.

CHAPTER 2

When is Less Insurance Better than More?

Why health insurance?

Understanding how health insurance works is the key to unraveling the Gordian knot of health care reform. Nothing will improve unless we fix the health insurance mess. Right now it covers too much, the wrong way, and doesn't sufficiently control costs. Health care reform should and must center on these issues.

Most Americans have health insurance coverage. Political rhetoric places access to medical care (and hence health insurance coverage) on the high pedestal of either a "right" or a "necessity." Yet food is clearly more important for people's lives and well-being than medical care. So, why does nobody worry about "grocery insurance"?

It almost sounds silly on the face of it—why would anybody insure against the costs of groceries? If we did so (as with health insurance) people would buy fine steaks instead of hamburger, and the most convenient types of semi-prepared food they could find. Breakfasts would consist of eggs Benedict and Belgian waffles, not a bowl of generic granola. National debates would fret about the cost of groceries.

Of course, the main reason we don't buy grocery insurance is that there's no real financial risk involved. Our grocery bills are very predictable in general, almost perfectly so, except for sporadic movements in the prices of fresh produce, meat, and dairy products. In the grand scheme of things, grocery costs are very stable and easy to manage in the household budget.

As a thought experiment, consider what would happen if humans' appetites varied wildly and unexpectedly from month to month. What if you suddenly awoke one morning and found that you needed to eat 25,000 calories per day instead of 2,500 to stay alive? What if, two months later, things returned to normal . . . and then suddenly, three years later, you found that you needed 250,000 calories a day to survive, and that lasted a month, upon which you returned to the normal 2,500 calories a day? If our bodies behaved like this, we'd probably all buy grocery insurance!

The point is that it's not the medical "necessity" that leads us to want health insurance. It's the financial risk imposed by highly variable health conditions from time to time. If medical events (and the costs arising from them) were as stable as our appetites and the subsequent grocery bills, none of us would want health insurance. People insure against risk and (most importantly) rare events that cost a lot when they occur. Illnesses (and subsequent use of health care) create just such a risk.

How health insurance changes medical care use

The unusual aspect of health insurance comes from the way it deals with the risk. We get paid for health "losses" *only* when we buy medical care. So the insurance distorts the choices we make, by lowering the price of medical care at the times we're deciding how much to use.

This turns the problem of designing an intelligent health insurance policy into a balancing act. We want to protect against financial risk, but at the same time we don't want to get sucked into a situation where we spend too much money on health care. After all, we (at least collectively) pay for the medical care we end up using through our health insurance premiums or taxes for governmental programs.

Insurance people call this problem a "moral hazard," a term arising from the situation where (as one example) some people might buy homeowners' insurance and then set fire to their homes to collect the insurance coverage. In health care, however, few people deliberately get sick in order to allow themselves to use their insurance. Illness and injury are not enjoyable. So in health insurance, the concept of moral hazard translates into the situation where people buy more medical care when they are insured than when they're not. If the moral hazard effect is small, designing good insurance is an easy task. With a large moral hazard effect, it gets more complicated; you need ways to protect against financial risk without encouraging the increase in medical care utilization too much. If we tip the scales too far, we get too much moral hazard overspending in exchange for only small improvements in risk protection. This is where "less" becomes better than "more."

The definitive study on how much this matters took place several decades ago, sponsored by the federal government and carried out by the RAND Corporation. It's known as the RAND Health Insurance Experiment (RAND HIE) (Newhouse 1993).[1] This study is still the gold standard in understanding how insurance coverage affects medical care use (and, to some extent, how that in turn affects health outcomes).

In the RAND HIE, participants gave up their own health insurance coverage while they were enrolled, and instead used a randomly assigned health insurance plan. All of the plans eventually had a "stop loss" feature, wherein all medical costs were covered after some threshold. But that threshold varied hugely across the plans. For some, the threshold was zero: full coverage for all medical care, no matter what. Their copay share was zero (copay = 0 percent).

---

1. In the spirit of full disclosure, I participated actively in the design and conduct of this experiment so, as one might expect, I think highly of its design and the veracity of the analysis.

At the other extreme, some families had an annual deductible representing a sizeable fraction of their annual incomes (5 percent, 10 percent, or even 15 percent of family income); for most medical events, they paid the full cost of their care, but they had catastrophic risk protection. There were also "in between" policies, those requiring families to pay 25 percent of their costs (copay = 25 percent) until they reached their catastrophic cap limit, at which time they too had complete coverage. Others had a 50 percent sharing rule (copay = 50 percent), and one group had an individual deductible equivalent in today's dollars to approximately $600 per person ($1,800 per family maximum) per year.

The easiest way to summarize the results shows the relative spending on medical care, compared with the full-coverage group (those who had completely free medical care). Figure 2.1 sets the utilization rates of the free plan (copay = 0 percent) at 100, and scales everything else in proportion.

The HIE analyzed much more than this table shows, but these categories of medical care give a good portrait of the wide set of results from the study. Insurance coverage matters in determining how much medical care people buy, but the effect is not all that large. At the extremes, the people with very large family deductibles spent 72 percent as much as those with full coverage, with the biggest changes in face-to-face medical (and related) visits (60 percent as much) and the smallest effect for hospital care (77 percent as much), as we might expect.

Two other interesting things appear in these data. First,

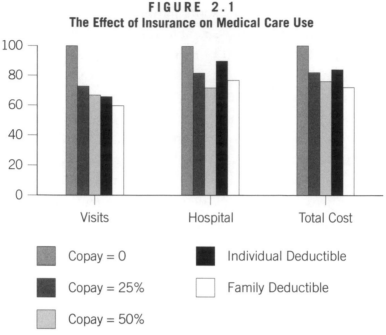

FIGURE 2.1
The Effect of Insurance on Medical Care Use

Legend:
- Copay = 0
- Copay = 25%
- Copay = 50%
- Individual Deductible
- Family Deductible

Source: RAND Health Insurance Experiment

paying "something" has the biggest effect of any change in coverage. Apparently, the step from full coverage (copay = 0 percent) to *any* payments by the patients gets the wheels turning differently. This is most obvious in face-to-face visits, where the consumer initiates the action.

Second, the individual/family annual deductible ($150/$450 then, equivalent to about $600/$1,800 now) had almost the same effect on limiting utilization as did a copay = 25 percent plan for care (up to the catastrophic cap the plans contained), but the simple deductible created much

36

less financial risk for individuals than an open-ended 25 percent copay program. It's pretty easy both to envision spending $600 (or $1,800 for a family) in any year on medical care and to budget for it. So an insurance plan with a significant individual deductible may be a pretty intelligent insurance plan both for controlling medical costs and for limiting financial risk.[2]

Controlling costs through provider incentives

It's clear from the RAND HIE results that consumer copayments help to control medical costs. But other mechanisms are available, too, most of which focus on health care providers. These fall into several groups: lump sum payments; case review/prior authorization; and pay for performance (P4P).

Lump sum payments: Lump sum programs pay for medical care in various prospectively defined clumps of care.

---

2. The federally authorized "Health Savings Account" insurance plans are somewhat modeled after this individual-deductible plan and family deductible plans from the RAND HIE. To qualify for the tax-benefitted HSA, the insurance policy must have an individual deductible of $1,200 (in 2010) with a maximum out-of-pocket expense of $2,400, after which all care is fully covered. HSA plans also incorporate a family deductible of $2,400, no matter what the family size, and an out-of-pocket limit of $4,800. Many HSA plans have a copayment such as 20 percent of all costs incurred between the deductible and the catastrophic cap limit, so (using this example), an individual would incur $1,200 in expenses below the deductible, another $6,000 in additional

These clumps might involve a fixed period of time (typically a year), or all of the medical care involved in treating a specific illness or injury (say, a hospitalization). They can be combined to involve, for example, the annual treatment for a single disease, such as diabetes. Let's review them in more detail.

Capitation: Capitation does not mean the grisly removal of a person's head (that would be de-capitation!), but rather the payment "per capita" for providing medical care for a fixed period of time, usually a year. The original capitation payment plans in the United States began in the Great Depression, including the Ross-Loos plan (founded in 1929) for employees of Los Angeles County and the Group Health Association of New York (1937). These were followed shortly by the Kaiser Permanente plans (1945) and Group Health Cooperative of Puget Sound (1947). We now call these types of programs health maintenance organizations (HMOs).

HMOs commonly show lower rates of hospitalization than their fee-for-service counterparts. Part of this comes from the incentives to avoid using the hospital, part comes from emphasis on preventive care, and part comes from favorable selection of relatively healthy patients into the insured pool. However, the RAND HIE compared a group of randomly selected patients in a large HMO with a comparable patient group given free care

___

expenses (leading to $1,200 out of pocket) and then would have full coverage.

(copay = 0) in the same city but in the more usual fee-for-service environment. The randomization eliminated the "favorable selection" aspect of the comparison. Yet, the RAND HIE found that the HMO enrollees were admitted to the hospital 64 percent as often as the "free care" fee-for-service counterpart group, and overall spent only 72 percent as much. Most of the savings came in the form of lower rates of hospitalization. Clearly, organizational structure and incentives play an important role in determining how much health care (particularly hospitalization) doctors recommend for their patients.

Case payment: The classic case payment model stems from a dramatic shift in the way Medicare paid for hospital services for the elderly. At its inception in 1965, Medicare adopted the standard approach for paying hospitals and doctors in private health insurance: fee for service. For hospitals, that meant that the hospital was paid for everything done for the patient—each day in the hospital, each hour of operating room time, each X-ray taken, each physical therapy visit, indeed, almost each bedpan cleaned. At the time, the emphasis was on access to care. However, burgeoning costs under the Medicare program soon led to a search for ways to control expenses. The first (and most successful) answer came in the form of a new way of paying hospitals: the "prospective payment" program now known as the DRG program.

Beginning in 1983, Medicare created hundreds of DRGs (diagnostically related groups). We now have about five hundred of them. They're based on the assumption that patients with similar medical diagnoses require similar treatment resources. Medicare developed an approved cost for treating patients in each DRG, and hospitals received that fixed amount no matter how long the patient was in the hospital or what services were provided.[3]

The incentive in this program is clear: find ways to shorten the length of stay, even if that requires use of other resources (such as more intensive physical therapy). This frees up the hospital bed for the possible admission of another patient. Despite the fact that hospitals do not have direct control over the length of stay (the attending physician, commonly a doctor in the community with hospital admission privileges, determines everything that happens to the patient, including discharge dates), hospital lengths of stay fell notably in response to the DRG payment system.

In the first full year before the DRG system, the average length of stay for Medicare patients was 10.6 days. At the end of the phase-in period, it was down to 8.5 days, reflecting an unprecedented 20 percent drop in length of stay. It was as if the United States suddenly had increased its hospital bed supply for the elderly (who account for almost half of all hospital admissions) by 20 percent without spending a dollar on new construction.

The DRG program was an unqualified success in

---

3. The program makes allowance for "outliers" with extremely long lengths of stay, but this applies to relatively few patients.

terms of its goals: Medicare saved billions of dollars over the subsequent years, and numerous analyses showed that (with few exceptions) patients were no worse off in terms of measurable health outcomes. Private insurance plans soon followed suit, and now most private plans pay hospitals on a DRG basis as well. Medicare also introduced reimbursement for alternatives such as hospice care through the years. Thus Medicare served as an important leader in finding ways to improve the incentives confronting health care providers.

To be sure, technical change has helped in this process through the years, most notably ambulatory surgery. But in some sense, the emergence of "one-day" surgery has made the reduction in hospital length of stay all the more remarkable, since many of the "easy" surgical cases are now done completely outside of the hospital in ambulatory surgery centers, whose patients don't get included in calculations of average lengths of stay in the hospitals. Nevertheless, we now see average stays for patients of all ages in community hospitals of only 5.6 days, versus 7.6 days in 1980, just before the DRG wave hit the hospitals.[4] This response represents another clear testimonial to the powerful effect of changing incentives facing health care providers.

Other uses of DRGs? If DRGs work so well for hospital admissions, why not use them to pay for other types of

---

4. The 5.6 day average would be even lower if we blended in the one-day stays of those receiving ambulatory surgery.

medical care? A careful look at the hospital DRG system shows why it's hard to move the idea to other types of treatment. The hospital admission has a well-defined boundary and purpose. The patient gets admitted for treatment of a specific illness or injury, often for a specific procedure (such as a particular surgical operation), and then returns home. Even thinking about paying the doctors involved in a single hospitalization makes little sense. A typical hospital admission could easily involve many doctors—the primary care doctor, a surgeon (perhaps with several assistants for a complicated procedure), an anesthesiologist, a radiologist (to interpret diagnostic images), a physiatrist (to oversee physical therapy), and perhaps a cardiologist to consult on the patient's fitness for surgery. Paying each of these doctors on a "per hospitalization" basis makes little sense, and trying to collect them into one unified payment has even more problems—who would receive the doctors' payment and decide whom to bring into the patient-treatment mix?

Carve-outs: Recent thinking about medical payments has created several new ideas, one of which combines case-payment and capitation. In this approach, patients with chronic disorders (e.g., diabetes, chronic obstructive pulmonary disease, asthma, or psychiatric disorders) have the treatments for their chronic disorders "carved out" for care by providers who get paid on a capitation basis. All other care for the patient can then come on a fee-for-service or separate capitation basis. The key goal is to get the chronically ill patient under the care of a well-trained specialist who best understands how to manage the disease in question.[5]

Mental health treatment sometimes gets carve-out treatment in current plans. Medicare is contemplating the use of carve-outs for people with chronic kidney disease. The range of chronic diseases where carve-outs might work is very broad and generally not well explored to date. Chapter Five discusses this issue in more detail, exploring the incentives of carve-outs for chronic care.

Case review: An entirely different set of cost-control measures employed by insurance plans doesn't use incentives, but rather has the insurance company peering over the shoulder of the doctors who actually treat the patients. The most common approach involves prior authorization.

In this approach, before the insurer will pay for expensive treatments (which can include hospitalization, expensive diagnostic tests, and elaborate dental treatments) the treating doctor must obtain approval from the insurer. To do this, the doctor (or, more likely, a registered nurse or other staff member) will contact the insurer in advance, describe the patient's condition and the need for the particular treatment, and sometimes engage in a ping-pong-like set of exchanges before the insurer approves the expensive treatment. Sometimes the proc-

---

5. This differs from disease management, which uses many of the same techniques, because of the bundled payment in a carve-out.

ess leads to a refusal to authorize the treatment. A "chilling effect" emerges where doctors may decide it's sometimes not worth the hassle to go through the authorization process, so they just don't offer the choice to patients. Thus, denial rates represent a lower bound on the effect of prior authorization plans on utilization.

I think it's fair to say that most patients and nearly 100 percent of doctors loathe the prior authorization approach. It interferes with doctor/patient decision-making, reduces doctors' autonomy, slows down patients' access to treatments, and adds costs—sometimes multiple staff members per doctor in the medical practice setting—to deal with the insurers. The problem is that we haven't found better mechanisms to control costs within the fee-for-service context.

Pay for performance (P4P): In P4P programs, the base compensation (whether fee for service or some lump-sum arrangement) is modified up or down as the provider exceeds or lags behind various quality targets. These quality targets can relate to specific treatments (e.g., case-mortality rate for heart surgery) or to wide goals for using preventive activity within a general practice setting. For example, a pediatrician's fees (set at 100 percent for a high level of compliance with the target) might take a 5 percent cut if the medical practice did not achieve at least 90 percent vaccination rates for children.

Two big problems stand in the way of widespread P4P. First, we don't have good performance measures in very many areas of medical care, and for good reason. It's relatively easy to set performance standards for "process" goals like vaccination rates. For diagnosis and treatment, it's much harder, because patients vary hugely in their underlying severity of illness and the extent to which they have co-morbidities (other illnesses that complicate the treatment). For example, those with angina often have diabetes and its associated problems. Figuring out how well a doctor, hospital, or clinic is treating patients with angina is greatly complicated by these other conditions and by variations in disease severity.

For these reasons, many performance standards don't look at health outcomes per se, but rather look at the processes of care—how often doctors (or health plans) undertake variously recommended preventive activities, how often they stay in compliance with various guidelines, etc. These process standards provide some guidance, but they mostly reward providers for doing specific things rather than for measurable improvements in their patients' health.

Many of the P4P incentive programs also use incentive payments that are too small to cause real behavioral changes. The incentive payments need to be large enough for the providers to invest in a real effort for change.

A second problem relates to the first one. All lump-sum payment programs and all outcomes-based P4P programs run this risk: if providers get paid a flat fee for treating a group of patients (e.g., capitation, DRGs for hospitals, etc.), and if the mechanism does not fully measure and capture all dimensions of patient complexity, then providers will have incentives to avoid, turn away, or transfer patients with unusually high risk characteristics. Without good risk adjustment in either lump-sum payment programs or P4P programs, patients with many complications, particularly those not measured in the programs' metrics, stand at risk of being set adrift with no provider willing to treat them.[6]

How much will people pay to avoid hassle?

Hassle-free health care is a true luxury. Many programs that promise to control health care costs involve things that both patients and their doctors view as an incredible hassle, most notably prior authorization reviews for expensive treatments. They can also involve gatekeeper

---

6. The history of Medicare Advantage Programs (Part C, sometimes called Medicare HMO) is littered with important examples of the problems of inadequate risk adjustment. In this program, Medicare enrollees can sign up for an HMO for all of their treatment, rather than using the usual fee-for-service system that Medicare was founded on. The difficulty immediately becomes apparent: if Medicare pays (say) the average cost in the region for treating a patient, the intelligently run HMO will try to attract relatively healthy patients and shun sickly ones. This happens at *any* level of payment so long as the payment does not vary with the individual's health condition. The trick becomes finding a way to measure the patient's likely *future* medical costs (and pay the HMO accordingly) in a way that makes the Medicare HMO not really care how sick the patient is.

programs requiring a primary-care doctor's referral before the insurance plan will pay for a specialist visit and, in a few cases, requirements for a second opinion before the plan will pay for treatment.

Another form of hassle arises in so-called Preferred Provider Organizations (PPOs), wherein the insurer strikes a low-price deal with providers, and then pushes patients (with incentives) to use those providers rather than other more-expensive providers (doctors, hospitals, pharmacies, etc.). The problem comes when the person's employer changes health insurance carriers (through bidding on the annual contract). If the employer changes carriers, the network of preferred providers also changes, often forcing patients to shift doctors.

Ongoing trends in the types of health insurance people select tell a simple story: when given the option, most people select lower-hassle plans even when they cost more. Gatekeeper plans, once a highly touted cost-control technique, have diminished in importance. Of course, when people opt for lower-hassle insurance programs, they're often doing it with "funny money" that doesn't cost them much. Chapter Four describes these issues more completely, with respect to both employer-provided insurance choices and the tax subsidy for health insurance. The tax subsidy almost surely leads many of us to have too much insurance, as Chapter 4 details.

CHAPTER 3

How Does Good Technology Go Bad? A Tale of Two Cities (and More)

The past several decades have seen amazing advances in science and technology that can improve our well-being (the good). These cost a lot of money, but they can bring great value—if used intelligently. Unfortunately, the ways these interventions get used in our society vary greatly, so we have some intelligent use and some wasteful use (the bad). Some comparisons of pairs of cities (such as Orlando and Miami, FL) show how much waste takes place in our system with over-use of some otherwise wonderful technologies (a "tale of two cities" and more). The incentives in our system don't promote intelligent use or help eliminate wasteful use, and this problem will persist until we find ways to alter these incentives (the ugly). Let's explore the good, the bad, and the ugly in more detail.

The good

Technological breakthroughs: Advances in imaging and surgery have transformed modern American medicine.

Diagnostic imaging: We've moved from blurry x-ray images to astonishing CT, MRI, ultrasound and PET scans, all of which can improve diagnostic certainty and hence improve health outcomes with amazing images of human tissues and organs.

Surgical improvements: New minimally invasive surgery (arthroscopy and laparoscopy) have greatly reduced the risks and disability from surgery and greatly shortened recovery periods. Improvements in anesthesia techniques have almost eliminated anesthetic deaths, which fifty years ago killed about one in 10,000 patients, and now only about one in 200,000.

Pharmaceuticals: Drugs have created immense gains in longevity and health over the past half-century or so, and we can expect even more in the future. Two of the great medical triumphs of the twentieth century involved antibiotics and treatments for mental illness.

Starting with the discovery of penicillin in 1928, sulfa drugs about the same time, streptomycin in 1943, and tetracycline in1950, antibiotics (coupled with clean water supplies) have almost eliminated deaths from infections in our country. In 1900, the death rate from pneumonia and tuberculosis was one per one hundred twenty five persons. Now it's one per one thousand seven hundred persons. Life expectancy increased by thirty years during the past century (from forty-seven to seventy-seven years), much of the gain coming from safe water and antibiotics. Antibiotics alone added eight years to life expectancy between 1944 and 1972.

In 1970, the United States had more than four hundred thousand inpatient mental hospital beds, a number that has now dropped below sixty thousand. Some of this shift in treatment came from the development of outpatient mental health centers, but much of it came with the introduction and refinement of psychoactive drugs. The results are remarkable: these drugs not only improved the health and well-being of patients with mental disorders, but actually reduced costs of treatment, primarily by eliminating hospitalizations.

Lyndon Johnson's other war: In addition to his major role in the Vietnam War and the War on Poverty, neither of which we won, President Johnson in 1964 created a commission led by famed heart surgeon Michael DeBakey, MD. The commission's report led to the "war" on heart disease, cancer, and stroke, the three main killing diseases of our time.[1] The results have been remarkable, while not yet a complete victory.

Heart Disease: As recently as 1980, heart disease accounted for over 38 percent of all deaths, falling to about 35 percent in 1990, about 30 percent in 2000, and near

---

1. The resulting legislation founded a set of Regional Medical Programs, a concept that lived only a decade, but the funding priorities established for NIH and other research remained intact, and the current NIH budget retains emphasis on these three sets of diseases.

25 percent now. This represents a remarkable reduction in death rates due to heart disease. How did this happen?

Certainly a significant part of the gain comes from reductions in cigarette smoking since 1965 (see Chapter Six), with smoking rates falling by half in the last half-century. Some also comes from the development of heart surgery, most notably coronary artery bypass graft surgery, and the more recent development of stents, small metal sleeves inserted into coronary arteries to help keep them open and clear for blood flow. The recent improvements mostly come from lipid-lowering drugs (e.g., statins), first marketed in 1987, which reduce deaths from all causes for people with heart disease by 20 percent (including a 35 percent reduction for heart-related deaths) and have beneficial protective effects even for relatively healthy people.

Cancer Survival: For all cancers diagnosed in 1975, the five-year survival rate (a standard indicator of successful treatment) was just 50 percent. The next two decades saw increases to 60 percent and then 66 percent.[2]

Some cancers have proven intractable. The pancreatic cancer five-year survival rate is only 5.2 percent (double the 2.6 percent rate three decades ago). Others have a high and growing chance of survival, including breast cancer (now 90 percent, up from 75 percent three decades ago), colon cancer (now about 65 percent, up from 40 percent in the sixties), and prostate cancer (up from

---

2. The data in this section come from the National Center for Health Statistics' SEER system (Surveillance, Epidemiology, and End Results).

69 percent thirty years ago to virtually 100 percent survival today for those diagnosed with anything other than widespread metastatic disease). Improvements in cancer survival have come from several areas, most notably improved early diagnosis (mammography for breast cancer and screening of various types for prostate cancer and colon cancer, for example) and improved chemotherapy and radiation therapy regimes.

Strokes: The third focus of Lyndon Johnson's health war—strokes—has also shown great improvement over recent decades, primarily due to newly discovered drugs. Stroke deaths fell by 40 percent between 1960 and 1980, stabilized for a decade, and then dropped another 25 percent since 1995. Some of this comes from reduced smoking, but much also from lowered hypertension and other risk factors—mostly attributable to new (and often widely advertised) pharmaceuticals.

What do we get for our money? Medical care has—on aggregate—a high degree of productivity in improving our health. The current debate about health care reform fixates on the costs of our health care system, often almost wholly ignoring the benefits. It's worth remembering how we benefit from our health care.

A recent analysis of U.S. mortality and medical spending data (Hall and Jones 2007) estimated the cost of adding a year of life to the U.S. population using current medical technology (see Figure 3.1). This analysis looks at medical spending rates and improvements in longevity, not at any specific treatment. It reveals in broad

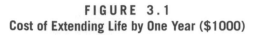

FIGURE 3.1
Cost of Extending Life by One Year ($1000)

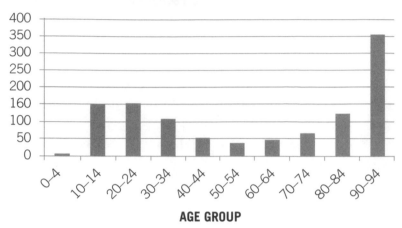

AGE GROUP

Source: Robert E. Hall and Charles I. Jones, "The Value of Life and the Rise in Health Spending," *Quarterly Journal of Economics*, 122:1 (February, 2007), pp. 39–72. Copyright ©2007 by the President and Fellows of Harvard College and the Massachusetts Institute of Technology

terms what we get when we spend money on health care. Hall and Jones only studied increases in life expectancy; hence, their work misses the many benefits of medical care that improve the quality of life (reduced pain, increased mobility, reduced anxiety, etc.) in addition to extending lives, so we can take this work as a lower-bound estimate of the benefits of medical spending.

As would come as no surprise to even the casual observer of the medical system, the results vary significantly by age. Saving the life of a young child (say, with a vaccine or newborn intensive care) adds many years of life, so we can expect the cost per life-year to be relatively low in that population, and it is: $8,000 per life-year saved.

We'd also expect that cost to rise for teens and young adults, since the primary causes of death in those age groups (vehicle crashes, other accidents, homicide, and suicide) usually involve expensive and complicated medical interventions. So we see costs per life-year saved rising to about $150,000 for this group.

We'd then expect the costs of adding a life-year to fall through middle age, the time when there are still many years of life remaining but our bodies have not aged so much that medical care has little effect. And those costs do fall, going down to $38,000 per life-year for ages fifty to fifty-five.

And finally, at very old ages, we should expect an increasing and eventually very high cost per life-year produced, because even if a single treatment is successful, the eventual consequences of aging take over. These costs rise rapidly, especially in the nineties and beyond, to more than $350,000 per life-year saved.

To put these data in perspective, look at Table 3.1, showing how the cost-effectiveness measures of various interventions differ depending on which group receives them. These show the costs per Quality-Adjusted Life Year— like the work of Hall and Jones but also counting gains for things like pain reduction and increases in mobility.

Consider the use of lipid-lowering statin drugs. In

TABLE 3.1
Estimated Cost-Effectiveness of Commonly Used Medical Interventions
(All Interventions Compared to "Usual Care"
Unless Otherwise Noted)

Intervention	Cost/Life-Year (2008 Dollars)
Low-Dose Lovastatin for High Cholesterol	
Male heart attack survivors, aged 55–64, cholesterol level ≥250	3,237
Male heart attack survivors, aged 55–64, cholesterol level <250	3,440
Female nonsmokers, aged 35–44	3,035,160
Female hypertensive nonsmokers, aged 35–44	1,436,631
Exercise Electrocardiogram as Screening Test	
40-year-old males	186,561
40-year-old females	502,826
Hypertension Screening	
40-year-old males	41,279
40-year-old females	63,333
Breast Cancer Screening	
Annual breast examination, females aged 55–65	22,865
Annual breast examination and mammography, females aged 55–65	61,512
Physician Advice about Smoking Cessation	
1% quit rate, males aged 45–50	5,666
Pap Smear, Starting at the Age of 20, Continuing to 74	
Every 3 years, compared to not screening	36,017
Every 2 years, compared to every 3 years	711,671
Coronary Artery Bypass Graft	
Left main coronary artery disease	13,152
Single-vessel disease with moderate angina	132,131
Neonatal Intensive Care Units	
Infants 1,000–1,500 grams	16,391
Infants 500–999 grams	115,742

Note: Garber and Phelps (1997, and citations therein), data converted to 2008 dollars using CPI.
Source: Alan M. Garber and Charles E. Phelps, "The Economic Foundations of Cost-Effectiveness Analysis," *JHE [Journal of Health Economics]*; 16:1(February 1997), pp.1–31, Copyright ©1997, reprinted with permission from Elsevier.

post-heart attack individuals, they extend lives at a bit over $3,000 per Quality-Adjusted Life Year (QALY[3])—a great bargain—but the same drug given to young, non-smoking women (at low risk for heart attack) costs $3 million per QALY. Similarly, Pap smears every three years add QALYs for women at $36,000 per year, but the added costs of increasing to every two years raises the cost per QALY to over $700,000 per year. Newborn intensive care units add QALYs at only $16,000 each, unless the infant weighs less than 1,000 grams, where the costs rise to about $116,000 per QALY. Many other examples abound.

As with the examples in Table 3.1, where the same treatment adds QALYs at highly different rates depending on the population treated, Hall and Jones show that the incremental costs of extending life by a year increase with patients' ages.

The costs per life-year also increase through time. The chance to pick the low-hanging fruit came earlier, e.g., through the use of antibiotics. To extend life even further now requires more complicated and expensive interventions. Hall and Jones estimate that the costs of extending life by a year have grown over the past half century at an annual rate of about 5 percent to 8 percent, depending on the age group. This closely parallels the annual growth rate in medical spending. Moreover, we can expect this trend to continue.

---

3. Pronounced "kwa-lee."

The future: New discoveries in the world of biological sciences suggest an even wider array of changes. With improved understanding of the role of genetic differences across individuals and how they affect disease and therapy, we stand on the edge of potentially amazing innovations in medicine:

- Possible cures for genetically linked diseases such as cystic fibrosis and other diseases such as some cancers
- Individualized therapy based on understanding how various genotypes respond to different therapeutic choices
- Refined searches for other therapies based on improved understanding of the biological pathways of disease mechanisms.

Innovations in "regenerative medicine" (based on stem cell research) hold the promise to reverse problems created by diseased or damaged tissue, including:

- Cure of neurological disorders such as Alzheimer's disease and amyotrophic lateral sclerosis (ALS)
- Growth of new bone and joint tissue to reverse arthritic damage
- Regeneration of pancreatic functions to reverse diabetes
- Repair of diseased portions of the cardiovascular system.

In parallel, a wide array of new bio-engineering inventions shows promise for improving human function. The past few decades have seen remarkable innovations in such areas as treatment of hip fracture; total joint replacement for arthritic or damaged knees, hips, and shoulders; vision improvement (lens replacement for cataracts and laser-guided vision correction); and continuous-injection insulin devices for diabetics. New artificial limbs have progressed to the point where a man with two artificial lower legs could meaningfully compete for a position on South Africa's regular Olympic track team in 2008.[4] The future shows even more promise, including such things as artificial retinas to bring sight to the blind, highly sophisticated artificial limbs, and artificial hearts.

These new medical and engineering discoveries can bring great benefits to our society, but we must be clear that few, if any, will lower health care costs. Most will cost more money, often much more. One of the great tasks of our health care financing system in the future is to devise intelligent and appropriate ways of introducing new technologies into the mainstream and assuring that they become available for those who will benefit sufficiently to justify the costs.

The bad

The bad news in all of this is that we don't have any good way of sorting out just who should receive various medical treatments and diagnostic interventions. The

---

4. He was so successful that some competitors claimed he had an unfair advantage from his prostheses, although none of them voluntarily had a leg removed and replaced with a similar prosthesis.

same thing occurs on a geographic basis. To put it mildly, our health care system demonstrates large scale confusion about whom to treat and how intensively to treat people. We see far larger systematic differences across geographic regions in treatment intensity than (on average) the difference in medical care use for those with no health insurance compared with those with excellent health insurance. One could write many tomes on the diverse practice patterns we find in the United States; here are a few examples.

A Tale of Two Cities (and More)

It's easy to find pairs of cities even within the same state that have radically different health care spending. The Dartmouth Atlas of Health Care (2009) has documented these regional differences in treatment costs, all adjusted for age and sex mix of the populations using Medicare data. The results almost verge on the bizarre.

Health care in Orlando, Florida, costs about half as much annually per person ($8,870 in 2006, the last year of complete data) as it does in Miami ($17,364). Miami's costs grew at 5 percent per year over the last decade, considerably above the U.S. average of 3.5 percent. Directly across the state on the Gulf Coast, Fort Myers ($8,366) and ritzy Naples ($8,125) come in even lower, and farther up the coast we find Tampa ($9,304) and St. Petersburg ($9,102) not much higher than Fort Myers or Orlando.

In New York State, Rochester ($7,916) costs 71 percent and Buffalo ($6,730) 61 percent of the cost of Manhattan ($11,008). In California, Los Angeles tops the charts ($11,981), yet San Francisco ($8,304), Stanford ($6,891), San Diego ($7,838), and posh La Jolla ($6,615) come in much lower. The "other" Rochester (Minnesota, home of the famed Mayo Clinic) has an average near that of other major metropolitan areas in the same state ($7,915 for Rochester, $7,092 for Minneapolis, and $7,406 for St. Paul).

Many other comparisons can be drawn from the Dartmouth Atlas data, but these examples make the point: regional styles dominate spending patterns, and the expensive styles cost vastly more than the average.

Further, broad-scale comparisons of health outcomes across the United States show that per-person spending has little to nothing to do with health outcomes. Those who live in the higher-spending areas don't live longer, they are not more satisfied with care, they don't have better functional status (mobility, freedom from pain, etc.); they just use more resources (Fisher, Wennberg, Stukel et al. 2003).

Further analyses of Orlando versus southern Florida have shed some light on how this happens (Skinner and Wennberg 2003). These regions differ only a little on treatments that generally exhibit low cross-regional variations (such as hospitalization for hip fracture, hernia repair, and the like) or for cardiac stent implants. A large part of the difference in per-person spending comes from the intensity of treatment, particularly in hospitalizations and intensive physician treatment at the end of life.

In another example, cancer specialists and urologists in Florida recommend prostate specific antigen (PSA) testing for prostate cancer for men over eighty at a much higher rate than the national average (67 percent versus about 40 percent), a practice widely believed to have little benefit for men of that age.[5]

The upscale spending patterns begin at the primary care level. Primary care doctors in high-spending areas are more likely to make specialist referrals, order more expensive diagnostic tests (even of minimal potential value), and recommend more frequent return visits. Even within a single region (and controlling for patient illness characteristics), doctors' styles can differ greatly in the costs of treating patients. Ranking total costs of care per patient of primary care doctors by practice style in Rochester, New York (a region relatively conservative in spending on average), showed that the patients of the top 10 percent of resource-users spent twice as much for care as the patients of the lowest 10 percent of resource users (Phelps 1992).

The ugly

The health care spending dilemma we confront in the United States has no single cause. In fact, it's pretty easy to show that the mess we're in requires a confluence of several things at once. One issue (the subject of the next

---

5. The U.S. Preventive Services Task Force specifically recommends *against* screening men over age 75 using the PSA test.

chapter) is the subsidy to employer-paid health insurance from our tax system. For those insured through this mechanism (a large fraction of those under age 65), this leads to insurance coverage that is overly generous, and in fact makes the costs of various treatment options essentially irrelevant to patients and their doctors. I understand that many people admire this feature of our health care system, but we must understand that this issue sits at the very core of the financial problems we face in the future, not only for health care but for the financial stability of our country.

Now, couple this overly generous insurance with the apparent confusion about how intensively doctors should treat patients. Completely setting aside issues of provider-induced demand (a topic of Chapter Five), it's clear that the lack of incentives for cautious spending combine in an unfortunate way with various practice styles.

Expensive treatment looming in my future? No bother! My insurance pays for it! Expensive practice style in my community? No bother! Our insurance pays for it! And relatively few individuals in the United States bear the full brunt of the effects on health insurance costs (or can't even see them) because of tax subsidies to insurance, because of hidden financing through employer-paid insurance mechanisms, or because Medicare does not alter the costs to participating in Parts A or B (the key parts of Medicare insurance) by region.[6]

---

6. Medicare Advantage (Part C) options—the HMO plans that Medicare patients can choose to enroll in—do vary in cost by region, as do Medicare Part D (drugs) insurance costs.

Making "the ugly" beautiful

What do we need to make more of the ugly become part of the good? No single solution exists. One thing does seem clear: fixing this problem requires some mix of incentives, information, and changes in insurance coverage decisions. All three of these have to improve for both providers and consumers.

Incentives: Incentives matter a lot in dealing with this problem. For consumers, we could change the ways in which insurance pays for care so that it continues to protect against financial risk but makes people more acutely attuned to the resource use they and their doctors decide upon. Current health insurance plans do this very poorly, and this offers a chance for significant change.

Patient incentives: Our health care system apparently operates with an almost overriding goal behind every decision: hide the true costs of care from everybody involved. Economists look at this and (to paraphrase the young star of the movie *Sixth Sense*) say, "I see hidden costs. They're everywhere. They don't know they're hidden."[7]

When we go to a doctor or an emergency room, or get admitted to a hospital, nobody talks about the costs of

---

7. Other nations also face these problems, but most have some sort of centralized budget cap to offset the other incentives, with a central authority having at least some understanding of the total costs.

various treatment options. Why not? In part because nobody has any incentive to know. The patients don't know or care. The doctors often don't know or care.

Recall how health insurance works (see Chapter One): you have to buy medical care to get any benefit from your health insurance (rather than cash payments for "events" like a burned home or crashed car that other insurance provides). The differences in incentives are very important. One gives us cash, the other reduces the price of medical care. The consequences (see Chapter Two) mean that those with the most generous insurance use about half again more health care than those with no insurance.

Some insurance gives you a good feel for the costs of care, but relieves you of much of the risk. Classic major medical insurance did this, and some of the insurance policies used today have this same feature. You pay for all of your care until you meet an annual deductible (say, $1,000 per person), and then the insurance pays 80 percent of your care until you hit an out-of-pocket cap, at which point the insurance pays 100 percent. These plans, currently known as high-deductible or consumer-directed health plans, reveal much of the true cost of care to the consumer for most illnesses and injuries, while also protecting against major financial risk.

Other insurance does everything possible to hide the cost of care from the patient. These plans either pay 100 percent of everything (a rare plan to find these days) or, more commonly, require a fixed payment of some amount (say, a $30 copayment) per doctor visit (with a higher amount such as $150 for a visit to an emergency room). The $30 cost applies no matter whether your doctor visit costs $60 or $600. The $150 emergency room cost applies no matter whether the total cost was $1,000 or $10,000. The consumer has no logical reason to bother finding out the true costs of care, and no incentive to think about finding a provider who might charge less. This type of insurance does almost everything possible to hide costs from the ultimate decision-makers—the patients and their doctors.

Americans tend to prefer plans that hide the costs: full coverage or flat dollar copay amounts for a visit. Partly, this comes from the tax benefit for employer-paid insurance premiums, an issue so important that I deal with it separately in the next chapter.

Provider incentives: For providers of health care—doctors, hospitals, dentists, nurses, pharmaceutical companies, etc.—many ways already exist to change provider behavior, ranging from hospital length of stay to the rates at which new drugs get into the marketplace. These also offer great opportunity for reshaping our health care system in desirable ways. Chapter Five delves into these issues in more detail.

Information: In many ways, what we face in health reform is a problem of information production and dissemination. Information is costly to produce and costly for providers and patients to acquire. Often, neither party has strong incentives to improve its supply of information. But therein lies one key to reforming our health care system successfully.

Provider information: Guidelines help physicians understand when (and when not) to employ a medical intervention. All physicians learn this art during medical school and residency training, as well as during their continuing medical education. But (as the widespread variability in medical practices across regions suggests) what they learn may differ greatly from what other doctors have learned in other settings. Too often, the teaching doctors' personal experiences guide their teaching recommendations. Systematically developed guidelines bring a wider range of experiences and, most important, systematic data (epidemiology and results of randomized controlled trials) into play.[8]

Researchers studying regional differences in medical practice intensity (read: cost) have found that where good practice guidelines exist *and* where treatment diagnoses are clear and treatment outcomes well understood, one finds little regional variation. The widespread resource utilization differences come in areas more subjective in diagnosis, less well understood in therapeutic consequences, and lacking in guidelines. Thus we have good reason to expect that more widely spread guidelines can help solve this puzzling problem of regional dif-

---

8. A physician friend once told me, "The most dangerous words you can hear a doctor say are, 'In my experience' . . ."

ferences in treatment patterns that do not match patient illness patterns.

Patient information: Patients can climb onto the information train just as can doctors. Individuals now have access to a dizzying array of information about medical treatments and their consequences through such diverse sources as the Internet, print media, and broadcast media. Each of these has its own strengths and weaknesses.

The Internet has numerous Web sites that articulate clear information about various medical conditions, such as WebMD and informational sites provided by numerous medical centers around the country. Many single-issue Web sites focus on a particular disease. Some are highly organized (American Heart Association, American Cancer Society), while others have more modest resources (e.g., Restless Leg Foundation, ALS Association, Muscular Dystrophy Association). Search engines lead patients to many such sites. Alas, the Internet also has numerous sites filled with incorrect information. That's the problem with the Web—it takes a knowledgeable reader to sort the wheat from the chaff.

Broadcast and print media now overwhelm us with "direct-to-consumer" advertisements, most notably for drugs that affect people's lifestyles, from hair loss remedies to the ubiquitous erectile dysfunction ads. But direct-to-consumer ads also cover drugs that can have important consequences for survival, including various cholesterol-reducing drugs (statins and their kin) and hypertension medications. These ads have been shown to increase patient awareness about such conditions, prompting them to initiate discussions with their doctors about the conditions and the drugs. What we don't know is whether these ads increase appropriate use more than they drive inappropriate overuse.

Insurance coverage decisions: How do insurance plans decide which treatments they'll cover and which they won't? The big gorilla in this area is Medicare. Many private insurance plans closely follow Medicare coverage decisions, so it's worth knowing how Medicare makes these choices.

The official Medicare language (built into the original legislation in 1965) says that Medicare will cover any treatment that is "reasonable and necessary." For decades, this language has precluded any meaningful consideration of the costs of treatment as part of the coverage decision. Through an elaborate process, Medicare now issues National Coverage Determinations regarding new treatments or technologies, often on the basis of what researchers describe as "fair or poor" evidence about the effectiveness and costs of the intervention. In some cases, coverage is granted only to people with defined severity of illness criteria (a small step in the right direction), but the Medicare process still falls far short of available evaluation and decision techniques.

A quite different (and arguably better) approach comes from the British National Health Service's (NHS)

National Institute for Health and Clinical Excellence (NICE), established in 1999. NICE's analyses span the range of drugs, medical devices, diagnostic tools, and the management of individual medical conditions. They consider both clinical effectiveness *and* cost-effectiveness in issuing their advice and regulatory rulings. They provide guidance on whether and how these clinical treatments and interventions should be used in the NHS, and also (like the FDA in the United States) assume a regulatory role to analyze safety and efficacy of drugs and medical devices. Unlike our FDA, however, they do not stop with "safety and efficacy" but often go on to carry out formal cost-effectiveness analyses that become part of the guidance about use of drugs and devices as well as some clinical interventions. Our health care system would be well served by adopting the same philosophy.

Why do we need to bring cost-effectiveness into coverage decisions into the US (both public and private insurance)? We need this because multiple incentives create a natural tendency to overspend on health care, and yet (unlike almost all other nations) we have no centralized force to counteract these tendencies. In our market-oriented system, coverage limits in both private and public insurance plans provide the best alternative. In addition, as the next chapter details, our tax system leads us to have too much insurance in general, further exacerbating this problem.

Summary

Our health care system behaves almost whimsically in terms of the way treatments get recommended and used. What treatment you receive (if any) may depend as much on where you live and what doctors you use as your actual illness or injury. Incentives and information for both providers and consumers of health care could help bring some rationality to this process, offering considerable opportunity for improving the effectiveness of our health care while controlling cost growth.

Several things falling into the "ugly" category are so ugly that they deserve special treatment. The next two chapters do just that. Chapter Four looks under the hood of the employer-paid health insurance process that sits at the core of the health insurance system for most Americans under age 65, a system propped up by a tax subsidy that distorts our choices and ultimately adds billions of dollars annually to our medical spending choices. Chapter Five looks at the incentives created in our health care system for patients and (mostly) providers. We can't make the system work better without understanding what the incentives lead to, and hence how to change them for the better.

CHAPTER 4

Why is the Employer-Paid Foundation of Health Insurance Riddled with Termites?

E mployer-paid insurance, the "foundation" of our private insurance system, is riddled with termites. The worst "termite" is the subsidy created by excluding employer-paid premiums from the income tax base, a subsidy that costs the government billions in tax revenue and (most importantly) leads us to have too much insurance. Employer-paid insurance coverage also limits choices of insurance for many people, causes some people to fear changing jobs, and forces some people (near the minimum wage) out of the labor force. All of these problems would vanish without the distortion created by the tax subsidy. So how did this happen—who let the termites loose in the foundation?

Almost by accident during World War II, the United

States enacted one of its most forceful decisions affecting the scope and cost of health care. Some companies seeking skilled workers in the face of a labor shortage (because of the demands of the military and other wartime efforts, and prohibited by government controls from offering higher wages), responded in typically ingenious American fashion by augmenting the (controlled) wages and salaries with (uncontrolled) health insurance coverage. This became a very popular fringe benefit during and after WWII.

The ad hoc rules of the WWII era allowed fringe benefits (including retirement and life and health insurance) to be exempt from both wage controls and personal income taxes up to 5 percent of wages. Post-war legislation capped the tax-free contributions of employers for life insurance, but in 1964 Congress codified the ad hoc rules to clarify that employer contributions for health insurance premiums remained exempt from taxation (Helms 2008).

A large fraction of workers in the United States, particularly those with incomes above the legally mandated minimum wage, have at least some health insurance coverage paid by their employers. About 40 percent of all workers have employers who pay the entire bill. On average, the Department of Labor estimates that about 80 percent of all health insurance costs come through employer payments. This arrangement, while convenient in many ways, distorts our health care system in many unhappy ways.

Many Americans (falsely) believe that employer-paid

insurance is "free" to them. Nothing could be further from the truth. In a competitive market society, at least in the long run, the cost of the "free" health insurance will be offset by wages lower than they would otherwise be.[1] This is increasingly true as the economy globalizes, because of competition from foreign workers putting downward pressure on labor costs. Economists have studied this for years, and conclude in general that a very large fraction (well over 90 percent) of the true cost of employer-paid health insurance falls on the workers. Employers pay lower wages than they otherwise would when they pay for health insurance. It's just a big, cruel joke to say otherwise.

A billion here, a billion there . . .

The numbers involved are large, even by federal budget standards. Repeal of the exemption would increase the taxable income base greatly while at the same time not distorting most people's incentives to work in any meaningful way. Current federal estimates say that the tax expenditures[2] on employer-paid health insurance for 2008

---

1. One caveat: if the worker's wages are at or near the legally mandated minimum wage, it's impossible to have wages fall sufficiently to offset costs of health insurance premiums paid by the employer. The consequence then is often a loss of jobs in the market rather than offsetting wages.

2. "Tax expenditures" are defined as reductions in tax revenue by legislative reduction in taxation rates (possibly to zero) on certain revenue categories. The largest three are exemption of contributions to re-

reached $226 billion, consisting of $133 billion in fore-gone personal income taxes and $93 billion of lost revenue to the Social Security Trust Fund (FICA taxes).[3] In 2008, total federal tax receipts from personal income taxes were $1.25 trillion, and the 2008 federal deficit came in at $450 billion, so the income tax expenditure on health insurance represents about one-tenth of actual personal income tax receipts and about one-quarter of the 2008 federal deficit.[4] The $93 billion loss to the Social Security Trust Fund represents 11 percent of the FICA revenues collected in 2008. All of these numbers will, of course, grow steadily through time.

How the tax subsidy distorts insurance choices

At the societal level, this represents more than a simple "tax expenditure." The first and biggest problem is that

---

tirement plans, lower rate of taxation of capital gains, and exclusion of employer-paid health insurance premiums.

3. Other estimates almost double this number (Helms 2008, Figure 2.5). This estimate includes standard "tax expenditure" calculations of the Joint Committee on Taxation, but also includes amounts not included in its earlier estimates. The difference centers on interpretation of Section 213 deductions (medical expenses above 7.5 percent of income). Earlier estimates presumed that disallowance of the employer premium payments would still allow individuals to deduct the costs under Section 213. The new estimates note (correctly) that full repeal of the exemption would not permit such a deduction under Section 213, hence increasing the estimated tax expenditure from earlier estimates.

4. The recession will cause much larger deficits for 2009, and probably 2010 and 2011. But the 2008 figure gives a reasonable (perhaps low) assessment of the steady-state story.

76

the tax subsidy distorts people's choice of health insurance. It costs (on average) about a third less than if the employer payments were taxed as income.[5] This subsidy (like any price reduction) leads people to choose more insurance than they otherwise would. In health insurance, this comes through choices like the general style of insurance (generous versus stingy), cost-controlling (such as HMOs) versus unconstrained, the extent of coverage of such things as routine dental care, and the size of deductibles and copayments.

These more-generous health insurance policies in turn affect people's choices of health care (see Chapter Two). Since people with more generous coverage use more health care, the tax subsidy to health insurance translates directly into increased spending on health care through more medical services consumed and higher prices.

While the magnitude of this effect is uncertain (re-

---

5. This estimate calculates the average of each taxpayer's marginal tax rate (MTR) and uses that to estimate each person's taxes saved by having income in the form of employer insurance payments rather than cash. Here's how the calculation works: the MTR is the proportion you pay of the next dollar you would earn. If you are in a 15 (or 22 or 28 or 33) percent federal income tax bracket, that's part of your marginal rate. But the complete MTR includes not only the federal income tax rate but also state and local income taxes, social security taxes (employer and employee contributions), and the 1.5 percent Medicare tax. The complete MTR averages to about 33 percent in the U.S. population (Congressional Budget Office 2005). If you get $1,000 as employer-paid insurance rather than cash, you save $1,000 times your marginal rate. So, on average, the tax subsidy saves people about one-third of the cost of their health insurance.

search on the effects of the tax subsidy on insurance choices is neither recent nor conclusive), the direction of the effect is clear: the tax subsidy increases total spending on medical care through the mechanism of increasing the extent and generosity of individuals' insurance coverage. Thus, the tax subsidy is part of the medical spending problem.

The second effect comes through the mechanisms to raise federal income tax revenues. If federal government rules reinstated employers' premium payments as taxable income, it would add about 10 percent to the tax base, which would allow (other things remaining the same) a reduction of about 10 percent in everybody's marginal tax rates. This could have strong effects on the overall economic activity of the country, since the relationship between marginal tax rates and national income and productivity is reasonably well known.[6]

Third, the presence of employer payments distorts decisions by firms about using overtime or part-time labor versus hiring new full-time workers. Mandating universal employer coverage (a key part of almost every univer-

---

6. Economists widely accept the notion that economic activity (measured by taxable income) expands when marginal tax rates fall. The debates center on how large the effect really is. If large enough, income tax revenues actually increase as tax rates fall (the Laffer Curve effect). Most current estimates suggest that the effect is not large enough to actually increase revenues with a marginal tax rate cut (Giertz 2009), but that's not the issue when the tax rate cut is combined with an increase in the tax base through elimination of the employer-paid insurance exclusion. If Congress were to repeal that exclusion, an appropriate cut in marginal tax rates and the expanded taxable income base would assuredly both expand tax revenues *and* increase economic activity.

sal health insurance proposal of the past half-century in the United States) would make this worse. If employers have to pay health insurance premiums for a new worker (even if working only half-time), they will sometimes find it cheaper to use overtime labor from existing workers who already have the health insurance cost built into the payroll or to hire several part-time workers with under-limit hours. This will occur more for workers at the low end of the pay scale, and most of all for those at or near the legal minimum wage. This process creates inefficiency in businesses' use of labor, particularly in situations where employer-paid health insurance is mandated by law.[7]

One obvious result (again, mostly for those at or near the minimum wage) is that unemployment will increase because of the differential cost of hiring new workers versus adding overtime labor for existing workers. Denying low-wage people jobs should not be a part of our national health policy, but that's what requiring employers to provide insurance to all workers does.

Effects on workers

At the individual level, employer-paid insurance also has some unhappy effects. One of these involves workers'

---

7. For example, a recent study of mandated insurance coverage in Hawaii found that employers shifted toward hiring employees for less than twenty hours of work per week, the cutoff for mandated insurance (Lee, Russo et al. 2009).

productivity and lifetime earnings; the other involves the degree of insurance choice available to individuals.

Job lock: The most sinister of these effects is the "job lock" created by health insurance. People with really good insurance at their current jobs don't want to take the risk of moving to other firms if they or somebody in their family has acquired a chronic illness. The insurance coverage at the new firm may find ways to exclude payment for prior conditions that moving workers bring with them.

The Health Insurance Portability and Accountability Act (HIPAA) of 1996 partly addressed this issue. The "portability" part of the rules (Title I of the act) sets limits on the extent that health insurance plans can refuse to cover pre-existing conditions. These rules did fix part of the problem, but loopholes and bypasses remain, and workers may not fully understand what might happen if they do move to a new job; just the fear of coverage exclusions may inhibit some workers from seeking more productive jobs.

The extent of this problem before HIPAA was considerable. The best estimate of the magnitude of the job lock showed that about a quarter of potential voluntary job changes that might have occurred did not because of job lock (Madrian 1994). Some of this effect will remain (if nothing else because of workers not understanding the new law and because of loopholes) so long as we have employer-paid health insurance.

Reduced choice: As Mark Pauly has pointed out (2010), using the tax subsidy through employer group insurance reduces the breadth of choices individuals have about their health insurance coverage. They get to choose among the small handful of plans offered by their employers instead of from the vastly larger array of plans available more broadly in the market. An individual (rationally) chooses an employer plan most of the time for two reasons: the tax subsidy helps pay for the employer plan, even if workers don't like it as well as what the "most preferred" plan might be; and if they stay in the same job and refuse the insurance, they won't get a raise from the employer to compensate them for the employer's reduced costs.

Dual-worker families have the option of having one worker at a firm providing health insurance and another worker taking full compensation in wages.[8] This option goes away with mandatory insurance through employment groups (or its equivalent—a penalty on firms not offering insurance coverage).

Removing the distorting tax treatment

What would happen if Congress reversed the 1964 ruling that exempts employer insurance payments from the tax

---

8. At Wal-mart, for example, about 20 percent of workers have coverage from spouses' insurance, according to Wal-mart data.

base? The entire story could be quite complicated, and would depend in part on what Congress did with the newly found income.[9] However, we can envision most of the broad strokes in advance:

- Employers would probably continue to offer group insurance as they do now. These groups offer a convenient basis for selling health insurance, and that remains broadly true even without the tax subsidy. They might even continue to pay for some of the premiums, although the incentives to continue doing so would diminish.[10]

- Some employees would opt for "no insurance" and take the money in income. This could increase the rate of people "going bare" unless the government required all individuals to have some health insurance (as states do with automobile liability insurance and banks do for homeowners). Most of the proposed health reform legislation in 2009 mandated individual coverage.

- Some workers would shop around for other types of insurance than that offered by their employers. Competition would increase employees' options on many dimensions of insurance.

- Most notably, perhaps with some time lags to reach a new equilibrium, consumers would generally opt for less-generous health insurance than they now hold.

---

9. The bulging federal deficit from the 2008 and 2009 bank bailouts and economic stimulus packages suggests the obvious answer—it's already been spent!

10. Firms may wish to do this even without the tax benefits to the extent that it contributes to a healthier work force, for example.

The last of these points is the most important. We have a nation that is simultaneously over-insured (those with the tax subsidy through employer insurance) and under-insured. The over-insurance comes naturally because of the price reduction from the tax subsidy. It's a basic law of economics; when the price goes down, people buy more.

The under-insured part is a more complicated story. Insurance markets sometimes work in strange ways, partly based on the inability of insurance companies to detect high-risk consumers. In auto insurance, the past history of moving violations and accidents provides a good clue about the future. In health insurance, the best predictors of medical costs in the future include family history, age, smoking history, and the presence of other chronic diseases such as diabetes. Insurance markets tend (when left to their own devices) to try to separate the sheep from the goats, trying to find ways to attract the (healthy) sheep and segment out the (unhealthy) goats in order to have them pay higher premiums.

Natural mechanisms that have evolved in health insurance markets help contribute to the high rates of non-insurance in the United States. Many of those without health insurance (to the surprise of many) turn out to be young, healthy, and employed. They are healthy "sheep" who've decided they prefer income to health insurance coverage, and they select employment accordingly. There are many others, of course, at the fringes of poverty who don't have insurance either, but the point is that the market segmentation arising from separation of sheep and goats contributes to the rate of people going without insurance.

It is sometimes (but not always) possible to make both the sheep and the goats better off by pooling the sheep and goats into a single pasture (to carry the analogy forward), despite the natural market proclivities to separate them (Phelps 2010). The goats are better off (for obvious reasons) by having the costs of their insurance go down. The sheep are *possibly* better off even if they end up paying for some of the costs of the insurance for the goats, because the insurance markets can get rid of the myriad mechanisms previously used to distinguish the sheep from the goats.

One obvious way to achieve this result is through government intervention in the market. But we also have a long history of a private and voluntary way of doing this—employer-provided health insurance.[11] Employers almost always treat every person in their insurance groups as equal in terms of how the costs of insurance are shared, even though (for example) it's clear that older workers cost the employer far more than younger workers, and larger families obviously cost employers more than smaller families. Yet no employer charges older worker more than younger workers or ten-person families more than three-person families for insurance. In

---

11. Note that it doesn't require the tax subsidy to have this happen. For example, employers (and many other groups) in Japan and Germany offer health insurance to employees without the tax subsidy.

these cases, it seems as if the employers and their workers decide that they are all better off by having the sheep and goats put into one "pasture" together.

Conclusion

The tax exemption for employer-paid health insurance (arising almost by accident during WWII and codified in the law in 1964) has had profound effects on U.S. health care markets. It has made the insurance of employed persons too generous—with the downstream consequences of higher medical spending than we'd otherwise have. It has also contributed (through the mechanisms of market equilibrium in the insurance markets) to the extent of the uninsured.

Doing away with favored tax treatment would not only reverse these unhappy economic consequences but would also add hundreds of billions of dollars annually to the tax receipts of the federal and state governments, allowing them either to help fund the growing federal deficit or to reduce marginal tax rates across the board to offset the increase in the tax base (or combinations thereof). It's an obvious step to take in any rational health care reform.

So why doesn't Congress take such a step? Vested interests (those with very generous employer-paid insurance) will lobby to block the change. The debate under way in late 2009 and early 2010 showed this clearly. The 2009 proposals would tax so-called Cadillac plans (those deemed highly generous) with an excise tax (levied at the insurance company level and passed along by market forces to consumers). Strong opposition appeared almost immediately to this concept from labor unions, which have long bargained for extensive (and expensive) health insurance coverage for their members. So taking such a step will require an act of political will that is difficult to sustain, particularly for any political coalition that depends heavily on organized labor for important political support.

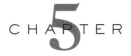

CHAPTER 5

Do Dollars Distort Doctors' Decisions?

Health care providers are human. They have multiple goals in life; they like to live in nice homes, take pleasant vacations, educate their children well, and . . . yes . . . they like to heal sick patients. Sometimes these goals come into conflict. How they behave depends in part on the incentives they face from regulatory agencies, insurance carriers, and, indeed, patients' own actions and decisions. Incentives also affect consumers' (patients') behavior. We saw in Chapter Two how health insurance changes patients' incentives. This chapter explores incentives that providers face and the distortion: arising there from.

How incentives matter

How doctors get paid matters. Many doctors are paid on a straight fee-for-service basis. The more they treat you, the more they earn. They need money to pay their office expenses, mortgages, golf club dues, college tuition for their children, and so on. So we can sometimes find situations where the way doctors get paid affects their recommendations.

This is a situation with no perfect answer. If doctors get paid more to do more, we can expect them to try to get some patients to use more medical care than they otherwise would. In the world of medical economics, we call this "induced demand." You encounter this in many other parts of life too. Sometimes it's very simple. Look at your shampoo bottle the next time you shower. It probably gives instructions on the order of, "Lather. Rinse. Repeat." You don't really need to "repeat." Once is enough. But if the manufacturer can convince you to repeat, it will sell you more shampoo.

Many people have taken a car in for repair and had the mechanic suggest an expensive repair job. Some people try another mechanic for advice. In medicine, we call this a second opinion. Sometimes the second opinion offers a cheaper way to fix your car. Sometimes the second opinion reveals that the first advice you got was pure fraud.

If this were the only issue, then we could readily prescribe that doctors be paid on a flat annual salary. But flat-salary compensation has its own problem: it reduces doctors' incentive to work hard, so that those supervising the doctors (e.g., more senior doctors in a group practice) have to make sure that they work diligently and intelligently (including not spending too much time with each patient). This problem becomes more difficult when the medical group is large and each doctor's mix of patients (each with his own illnesses and complaints) may require different amounts of time. One careful study of medical practices (Gaynor and Gertler 1995) showed that doctors on a full fee-for-service system worked longer and saw more patients per hour than those on salary, and the monitoring effect also showed up clearly. On average, the salaried doctors in large groups (at one end of the spectrum) had about half the productivity of the doctors in a fee-for-service arrangement.

The optimal way to pay doctors probably would have a blend of salary and fee-for-service. It's somewhat like car sales agents. Some are on full salary, and they don't pester you much when you walk in the car showroom. Some receive a smaller salary and get much of their income on commissions. They tend to be *very* attentive when you walk in the door . . . sometimes more than you wish. The optimal blend of salary and fee-for-service payments for doctors has yet to be figured out. Most doctors get paid one way or the other, but not a blend.

Some examples of induced demand

A vast literature has grown up during the past decades as health economists have tried to measure the extent of induced demand and understand its consequences. The conclusion is about what we could expect in a situation where one party (the doctor) knows a lot more than the other (the patient): we find evidence that demand inducement occurs, and that the extent of it hinges on the incentives and the rules of the game. The following examples illustrate the concept of demand inducement.

Caesarean section rates: The decline in birth rates over the past several decades has squeezed the business of obstetricians a bit. With fewer births, they have fewer babies to deliver. It's hard to talk people into having more babies just so the doctor can get another fee for the delivery, so we don't anticipate much induced demand on that front. But there's another aspect of the delivery that does admit the possibility of induced demand— whether the doctor recommends a Caesarean section or a vaginal delivery. Insurance plans pay more for C-sections than for normal deliveries. In addition, C-sections can be scheduled in advance, cutting down the inconvenience of 3:00 a.m. deliveries. Gruber and Owings (1996) took advantage of the fact that birth rates declined at different rates over time in different states. Thus the state-by-state data on births and C-sections provided a natural experiment on the question of how much doctors change their advice when facing declining incomes.

The answer is, "It matters, but not a lot." Over a decade-long period when overall birth rates fell by 14 percent, the speed of decline differed from state to state. Using these data, Gruber and Owings could estimate that a drop of 10 percent (relatively) in birth rates led to an increase of about 3 percent in the rate of C-sections. While other issues may affect these results, this provides (along with many other similar analyses) evidence of modest demand inducement.

Payment for surgery: Medicare changed the reimbursement schedules for doctors in 1990 with the intent of compensating doctors more or less the same amount of money per unit of time worked (with adjustments for complexity), a shift that was widely expected to reduce incomes of surgeons and other procedure-intensive doctors and increase incomes of "cognitive" doctors (primary care, etc.). One analysis of Medicare data (Nguyen and Derrick 1997) showed that the doctors facing fee reductions with fee schedule changes in Medicare had volume increases to offset about 40 percent of their fee losses, while those not facing fee reductions did not change their behavior.

Another analysis focused on thoracic surgeons, who were predicted to lose about a quarter of their income from the Medicare fee changes if surgical volume remained the same. This work showed that 70 percent of the anticipated decline in incomes was offset by volume increases by the thoracic surgeons, both Medicare and private patients alike (Yip 1998).

Own-your-own diagnostic facility: When you get an x-ray image, MRI, CT or PET scan, two different bills show up at your insurance company (or in your mailbox,

91

if you're not insured). One comes from the doctor who interpreted the image—the radiologist. The other comes from the facility that owns and operates the imaging equipment. Sometimes it's a hospital in your community. Sometimes it's a group of radiologists who invested in their own equipment and building. Sometimes the doctor who treats your illness or injury owns the equipment. Having a stake in the imaging facility obviously changes the financial consequences of your doctor referring you for an imaging study. Although such ownership is not very common in some states, it happens quite often in others.

One study (Hillman et al. 1990) analyzed data from 65,000 insurance claims to study how often doctors (such as orthopedic surgeons) referred their patients for imaging studies in two cases—those where the doctor had an ownership stake in the imaging facility, and those where the doctor didn't. This turned out to matter a great deal: those doctors with a stake in the imaging facilities recommended imaging studies at *four times* the rate of similarly trained doctors who did not own imaging facilities.

Therapy referrals: A similar analysis (Mitchell and Scott 1992) of doctors' recommendations about the use of physical therapy showed the same types of results, albeit with a much lower magnitude. Physicians who had a stake in physical therapy recommended 39 percent more therapy than those who didn't; and the licensed physical therapists in physician-owned facilities spent about 60 percent more (billable) time with patients than those in independent facilities.

Drug prescriptions: Doctors in the Old West wandered from town to town, carrying their medicine stock with them in a wagon. They were their own pharmacies. Some doctors got a reputation for being quick to recommend a particular salve or balm. They were called "quick-salvers," which soon became shortened to "quacks." That's why we call dubious doctors "quacks."

Modern medical ethics and laws ban doctors from dispensing drugs in their offices. The reason for this concern is obvious after we've read about imaging and physical therapy. We'd expect that if doctors sold prescriptions out of their offices, they'd end up prescribing a lot more drugs than they do now.

We have an interesting cross-cultural comparison of the same phenomenon. Despite widespread attempts to curtail or ban the practice, doctors' offices and clinics in Japan commonly sell medications to their patients, despite a law passed by the Diet in 1955 to separate prescribing and sales of drugs (the law is riddled with loopholes). It may come as no surprise to the reader by now to learn that the Japanese population is the most highly medicated in the world. A careful study of Japanese medicine showed that the average Japanese adult gets 20 prescriptions per year. In the United States, the comparable figure was about half of that.

A randomized controlled trial

As my students in health economics have come to learn, I have a great affection for randomized controlled trials as the gold standard for evidence about causation. It turns out that we have such a trial on the effect on demand inducement of compensation schemes for physicians (Hickson, Altemeier, and Perrin 1987).

In this study, a group of pediatric residents was randomized to receive either a flat annual salary (as is common for doctors in training) or a fee-for-service arrangement (as is common in the medical practices to which they would move after they completed their training). The pay was for services the residents provided in the teaching hospital's free-care clinic. The fee schedule was set so that, on average, each doctor would receive about the same annual income, no matter which payment mechanism applied to them. Of course, the doctors on salary had no incentive to increase visits from their patients (children, accompanied by a parent), whereas the doctors paid on a fee-for-service basis could earn more money by having their patients return for more follow-up visits. The patients were also randomized to even out the illness burden of each doctor's patient load.

An important aspect of this project was the role of "well-care" visits for the children—preventive checkups, vaccinations, etc. All pediatricians know the schedule of recommended well-care visits for children at every age; it's as much a part of their knowledge base as is human anatomy. So in this study, the authors could see not only what happened to recommendations about visits for the children, but also how the doctors performed relative to the well-care schedule set by the American Academy of Pediatrics (AAP).

Briefly, the fee-for-service doctors saw each of their patients on average about one more visit per year (about five instead of about four visits per year). Almost all of the increase in patient visits occurred in the "well-care" category, with no meaningful distinctions for more acute illness visits. This is just as one might expect from the economic incentives these doctors faced. Those paid by fee-for-service recommended more for their patients . . . and the children's parents complied, bringing their children back for the extra visits.

Behavior relative to the AAP standard is also illuminating. Again, the fee-for-service doctors were more likely to meet (and occasionally exceed) the AAP well-care recommendations. The salaried doctors fell back—not much, but some—below the AAP recommendations. This also accords directly with the economic theory, since these doctors would receive no extra pay for extra visits; indeed, any extra visits would cost them valuable time.

The bottom line here is that there was a modest amount of demand inducement—probably not enough to categorize as crucial, but nevertheless informative. We would be remiss, of course, in extrapolating the *extent* of demand inducement found here to other settings, but this represents about the strongest possible evidence that the economic concept of demand inducement is alive and well, even among generally altruistic pediatricians.

Introduction of new technologies

The process of bringing new drugs, medical devices, and medical procedures to market involves a wide array of legal and regulatory issues. The steps involve incentives for discovery and invention (both private and public); the regulation of medical drugs and devices (safety and efficacy) and testing to satisfy these regulations; the ways in which insurance policies include drugs, devices, and new medical procedures in their insurance coverage packages; and the ways in which the manufacturers advertise their products (both to providers of health care and directly to consumers).

This begins with the way NIH budgets are set. Although much of the research budget leads to very general and often very basic biomedical research, targeting and focusing those funds can shift the priorities of researchers around the country. The successes we have had with heart disease, cancer, and stroke come in part from priorities set in the 1960s. NIH-funded research provides extremely valuable building blocks for drug and device manufacturers as they take that basic research and turn it into marketable products.

Next comes the intellectual property law, where our patent law increasingly shifts to conform with international law. For drugs in particular, but also for medical devices, we live in a global economy; but all drugs and medical devices sold in the United States must conform to U.S. rules, no matter where they are made. That law provides for a twenty-year patent life, but FDA-required testing makes the usable patent life closer to a dozen years than twenty. Those rules require that the manufacturer demonstrate, eventually with large clinical trials, that the drug is safe (or that the benefits outweigh the risks) and actually improves health ("efficacious"). Once a patent expires, other manufacturers can enter the market with generic substitutes using the same chemical formula, usually at lower prices than the original product.

Pharmaceutical and medical device manufacturers have for many decades advertised their products heavily to the medical profession, with ads in medical journals, booths at professional meetings, and armies of sales representatives visiting doctors in hospitals, in the doctors' offices, and elsewhere. More recently, as noted above, we have seen the addition of direct-to-consumer advertising in print media and on television.

The final step in this process involves decisions by insurers about covering drugs, devices, and medical procedures. As noted previously, the major player here is Medicare, but numerous large private health plans make similar decisions for every new drug, device, and treatment option. Medicare has generally not considered cost (or cost-effectiveness) in its decisions, an issue that remains outside the current legislative debate. Most private plans will not cover "experimental" treatments, so individual coverage decisions sometimes hinge on when a treatment shifts from experimental to routine.

Every step along the way involves different incentives. The ways the NIH pays for research alter the types of research done in medical schools and research centers. Patent law creates incentives for drug and device makers. FDA rules alter those incentives through the costs of required safety and efficacy testing and the time involved to complete those studies—time is of the essence in many drugs. FDA rules also affect advertising strategies for drug companies, which in turn alter the costs of acquiring information for providers and consumers. Finally, insurance companies in turn create incentives for doctors and patients to use (or not use) a new medical drug, device, or treatment strategy through coverage decisions. These range from "yes/ no" coverage decisions to decisions about what "tier" a prescription drug plan might place a particular drug in, and hence the copayment required of the patient.

A big problem that needs new incentives: chronic care

Patients with chronic illnesses dominate our health care system. Yet, the payment system we generally rely upon (fee-for-service medicine, made worse by generous insur-

98

ance) seems almost perfectly designed to create treatment patterns for those with chronic illnesses—particularly those with multiple chronic conditions—that produce bad outcomes and very high costs. This is partly due to specialization in medicine: specialists, particularly those who do expensive procedures, earn much more per year than those who merely think and talk with their patients. Concerns about malpractice lawsuits probably don't help either. ("Hmm," says the general medicine internist, "that's a little out of my territory . . . why don't you see Dr. Goodliver for the cirrhosis problem and Dr. Wiseheart about the palpitations?")

The care of these patients becomes fractured; often, no single doctor can even list all of the patient's illnesses, and none is qualified to treat them all. Thus the care often badly lacks coordination, so we can find patients seeing one doctor to relieve symptoms that are the side effects of another doctor's prescribed drugs. Sometimes the drugs interact badly, sometimes fatally. Recent estimates say that one in twenty-five elderly Americans take combinations of drugs that put them at risk for drug-drug interactions (Qato, Alexander, Conti et al. 2008). Patients with multiple chronic illnesses can have more doctors than they have fingers.

This issue *really* matters. According to an analysis following a group of U.S. citizens over time (Anderson 2004), people with chronic conditions account for 85 percent of all health care costs. That's not a typo: 85 percent.

TABLE 5.1
Number of Chronic Conditions

	0	1	2	3	4	5+
Percent of all Medical Costs	15	20	18	14	12	21
Percent of US Population	51	23	12	6	4	4
Costs relative to person with no chronic conditions	1	3	5.2	7.9	10.3	23.4

Data source: Anderson, 2004

The problem accelerates as the number of conditions expands. Table 5.1 shows the extent of the problem. As the final row shows, those persons with five or more chronic conditions use twenty-three times as much medical care as those without any chronic conditions. Figuring out how to deal with chronic illness is one of the most important issues facing our health care system.

The problem will loom even larger in the future: the frequency of chronic conditions rises rapidly with age, and the aging of the U.S. population will make multiple chronic conditions more and more prevalent.

The other scary part about this is that most of these chronic conditions occur much more often in overweight and obese people (heart disease, hypertension, osteoarthritis, diabetes mellitus, and many others), the frequency of which is increasing rapidly in our nation (see Chapter Six). So the problem of chronic diseases will get worse and worse unless we radically change the way we treat such people. Finding the right incentives and support systems for patients dealing with these lifestyle choices will be a big part of dealing with the chronic illness problem.

In concept, we know how to deal with the incentives for these issues, but implementing them will take careful research and political will. Part of the problem involves changing patient behavior and part of it involves the way the health care system deals with people with multiple chronic conditions. Fee-for-service mechanisms seem almost doomed to repeat what we've seen in the past, reminding us of a comment often attributed to Albert Einstein: insanity is doing the same thing over and over and expecting different results. They almost guarantee fractured, uncoordinated care.

The most useful approaches to helping people with multiple chronic conditions will probably use "bundled payments" of some sort for treatment. With this approach, for example, a group of providers receives a lump sum for a year to treat a patient with chronic condition X. The providers then have incentives to find lower-cost approaches to treating the patient (such as involving nurses, social workers, and home health aides), avoiding drug-drug interactions, and, most of all, finding ways to keep the patient healthy enough so that hospitalization is not necessary. Almost everyone familiar with these issues understands that coordinated care with non-physician help in addition to the physicians pays off.[1] These programs are called "carve-outs" since the care for the

---

1. This goes beyond trained health care personnel. For example, in Britain, when somebody returns from the hospital with a condition that limits mobility, a carpenter comes to the home to assure that appropriate ramps and other assistance devices will help the person retain independence.

chronic illnesses gets separated from the care for other acute illnesses and injuries.

But this path has many shoals upon which good intentions can crash. First of all, the issue obviously becomes more complex for patients with multiple conditions. This is very common: of those people with any chronic conditions, over half have more than one. Getting the right bundled payment obviously grows in complexity for those with multiple conditions.

Second, and perhaps more important, is that people with the same diagnostic label (e.g., asthma, hypertension, diabetes) may bring very different medical problems to their healers. This brings the problem of risk adjustment to the foreground. Unless the categories for payment have appropriate fine-tuning, providers will shun those who seem to have overly complex conditions, since it will cost more to care for them than the average payment provides.

This is another complex incentive problem. *Any* single flat fee to providers for caring for chronic care patients will cause this sort of behavior: seeking out relatively healthy patients and shunning relatively unhealthy patients. The only way to prevent this is to sufficiently fine-tune payments (matching the patients' expected costs) to the point that the providers don't care much about an individual patient's degree of illness.[2]

---

2. In Medicare hospitalizations, a hospital is paid a lump sum for the entire hospitalization event, but Medicare now has about 500 diagnostically related groups (DRGs) that have similar degrees of patient severity. Lump-sum payments for chronic diseases may need the same degree of fine-tuning to make such a system work.

A patient incentive problem occurs when patients fail to fill their prescriptions regularly, sometimes skipping days of pills to save costs. The problem is that the drugs won't work if not taken regularly. So we need to think about the right way to get patients to buy and take their drugs, perhaps providing them at no cost, and maybe even rewarding them for taking them daily.

Summary

Doctors, like other humans, respond to incentives. One of the ways they do this hinges on the vast differences between doctors and their patients in their knowledge of health conditions and treatments. We go to doctors because we expect them to know more—much more—about how to treat our illnesses than we know. Thus we go to the doctor pretty much with the presumption that we'll accept any recommended treatment. So when doctors' incentives change—from reduced demand for their services, changes in reimbursement rates, or ownership of facilities—they sometimes change their recommendations. This doesn't occur very often (except for a few situations such as ownership of diagnostic imaging facilities) but it happens often enough to assure us that we need to pay attention to those things in designing an intelligent health care system.

Finally, chronic care treatment—likely best accomplished by using bundled payments for the entire scope of treatment for chronically ill patients—creates a whole array of incentive problems, ranging from those for patients (lifestyle choices and their effects on health outcomes) to the incentives to acquire and use prescription drugs regularly. But we really don't know how to do these types of programs well.

On that note, I turn to the most pressing problem of our long-term health outcomes and health care costs—the lifestyle choices Americans make and their effects on health.

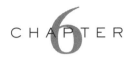

CHAPTER 6

Why Are We Killing Ourselves?

Most people in the United States don't understand the true causes of death. We read about deaths from heart disease, cancer, and stroke, but these are just the natural consequences of the true causes. The hard, cold truth is that our own choices are the primary causes of illness and death.

In a powerful study combining epidemiologic studies and mortality data, two researchers (McGinnis and Foege 1993) looked at the "excess mortality" arising from various lifestyle choices and combined that with death certificate data to come to an astonishing conclusion: the leading causes of death in the United States are . . . ourselves!

To see how this works, think about Disease X. Suppose that last year, one thousand people died of Disease X. That's what would show up in death certificate data. Now

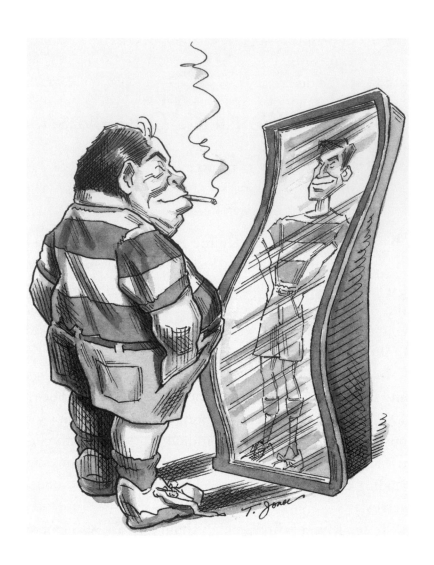

suppose that of those one thousand people, eight hundred were tobacco smokers. Since only about 20 percent of the U.S. adult population smokes, tobacco users are over-represented among those who died of Disease X by a factor of four. If the disease were unrelated to tobacco use, we'd expect to find only two hundred tobacco users among the one thousand who died of Disease X, but we actually saw eight hundred. So we attribute six hundred "excess" deaths from Disease X to tobacco.

Now do the same thing for other diseases, such as the real diseases of lung cancer, many other types of cancer, chronic obstructive pulmonary disease, heart attacks, heart failure, strokes, etc. Then add up the excess deaths attributed to tobacco. When you finish that list, it turns out that tobacco is the leading cause of death in the United States. The original study was redone ten years later using data from 2000. What was found is shown in Table 6.1.

This is pretty stunning stuff. These nine causes of death account for about half of all deaths, and most of these—surely we would include tobacco, diet/inactivity, alcohol, motor vehicles, firearms, sexual behavior, and illicit drug use—are wholly matters of human behavior and choice. One could easily include toxic agents (primarily consequences of air and water pollution) in the list as well, but that may be more of a societal than an individual choice issue. Let's look at the biggies in a bit more detail.

TABLE 6.1
Actual Causes of Death in the United States in 1990 and 2000

Actual Cause	No. (%)ᵃ in 1990 ᵇ	No. (%)ᵃ in 2000
Tobacco	400,000 (19%)	435,000 (18.1%)
Poor diet/physical inactivity	300,000 (14)	400,000 (16.6)
Alcohol Consumption	100,000 (5)	85,000 (3.5)
Microbial agents	90,000 (4)	75,000 (3.1)
Toxic agents	60,000 (3)	55,000 (2.3)
Motor vehicle	25,000 (1)	43,000 (1.8)
Firearms	35,000 (2)	29,000 (1.2)
Sexual behavior	30,000 (1)	20,000 (0.8)
Illicit drug use	20,000 (<1)	17,000 (0.7)
Total *(these 9 causes)*	**1,060,000** (50%)	**1,159,000** (48.2%)
All other causes	1,060,000 (50%)	1,246,000 (51.8%)

Notes: ᵃ The percentages are for all deaths.
ᵇ Data are from McGinnis and Foege.
Source: Modkad et al., "Actual Causes of Death in the United States, 2000," *JAMA*, March 10, 2004, Vol. 291, No. 10, 1238–1245. Reprinted with permission. ©2004 American Medical Association. All rights reserved.

Tobacco Use

Despite the enormous mortality burden from tobacco, the problem is actually declining. Some of this comes from improved cancer treatment (arising from NIH research in part). Much of the improvement comes from reduced smoking rates. Americans now smoke at about half the rate that they did in 1965.

Many things converged to cause this sea change. The most important was the Report of the Surgeon General of the United States on smoking, issued in 1964. Figure 6.1 shows what the per-adult cigarette consumption patterns look like.

FIGURE 6.1
Tobacco Consumption per Capita in Past Century

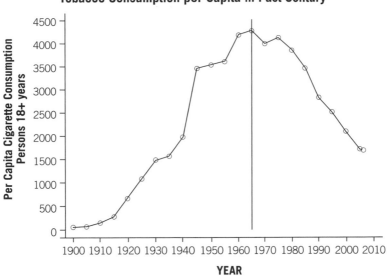

Data source: Health United States, 2009, US Department of Health and Human Services, National Center for Health Statistics, Hyattsville, MD, 2010, Table 61.

The transformation beginning in 1965 came directly from the 1964 Surgeon General's report and the many cultural and legal changes that followed.[1] Warning labels appeared on cigarette packages. Congress banned TV ads for tobacco, and numerous anti-smoking ads were

---

1. Other factors come into play also, including income and cigarette prices. So do wars. We all know that war is bad for people, but in addition to standard wartime casualties, we need to add smoking-related deaths. As Figure 6.1 shows, smoking rises dramatically during wars, especially WWII, when the Red Cross (and others) gave away cigarettes to soldiers.

aired. Local and state governments banned smoking in restaurants. Federal rules prohibited smoking on airplanes and local governments banned it in most airports. Cigarette taxes increased dramatically. Cultures changed. Before the Surgeon General's report, cigarette smoking was a standard Hollywood sign of sophistication. Ayn Rand praised smoking extensively in *The Fountainhead*. Now the public perception of smoking is quite different.

The Surgeon General's report—a compilation of known risks from the available medical literature—initiated a major change in smoking behavior in the United States. Instead of almost half the adult population smoking cigarettes, now under 20 percent does so. Luther Terry, MD, who was Surgeon General from 1961 to 1965, probably saved more lives than any other physician in history, simply by convening the committee that wrote *Smoking and Health: Report of the Advisory Committee to the Surgeon General of the United States*.

Eschewing the fat

Poor diet and lack of exercise make it to Number Two on the Hit Parade. With falling death rates from cancer and reduced smoking, this factor will soon reach the top of the charts. I know this is politically incorrect to say, but I'll say it anyway: FAT KILLS. Being overly skinny is also unhealthy, but that's not the problem we have for most citizens of the United States.

The Body Mass Index (BMI) is widely used to measure obesity, defined in metric measurements as weight in kilograms divided by height in meters squared.[2] I weigh 203 pounds (92.3 kilograms) and am 71 inches (1.80 meters) tall, so my BMI is 28.5.[3]

Numerous BMI charts and calculators are found on the Internet. Standard definitions put normal weight for adults as a BMI between 22 and 24, overweight as 25 to 29, obese as 30 to 35, and over 35 as morbidly obese. A large and growing fraction of the U.S. population falls into the obese and morbidly obese categories. We have an epidemic of obesity in the United States (and around the world), yet it draws far less attention than do many far less dangerous epidemics of various "bugs."

First, let's look at the data on the growth in obesity. Figure 6.2 shows data from a regular survey of the U.S. population from 1960 onward. Around 1975, the proportion of the U.S. population that was overweight (BMI > 25) started to grow. Almost all of the growth (see the third line down in the graph) comes from increases in adults who are obese (BMI > 30). The same general trends appear in younger age groups, too.

Now let's look at the effects of obesity on health. First, consider the ultimate indicator of health: survival rates. Figure 6.3 shows the relative risk of death in any single year by BMI category, separately for men and women of

---

2. To use imperial measurements, use weight in pounds, height in inches, and multiply by 703 to correct for the differences between the measuring systems.

3. To further add complexity, a new path of research suggests that waist circumference or the ratio of waist to hip circumference may explain all-cause mortality better than BMI—but let's not confuse the issue here with the specific measurement technique.

FIGURE 6.2
Obesity Trends in the United States

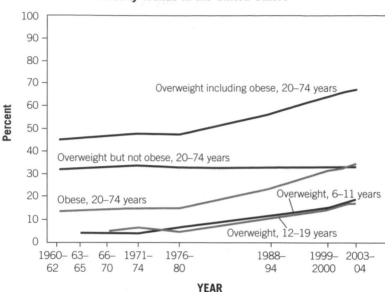

Data source: Health United States, 2009, US Department of Health and Human Services, National Center for Health Statistics, Hyattsville, MD, 2010, Figure 7.

ages 35–89 using the lowest-risk group as "1." Thus a relative risk of 1.5 means a person has a 50 percent greater chance of dying than a person in the best BMI group. These data show the risk relative to the lowest-risk group (females with BMI in the 22.5–25 range).

These data come from a "meta-analysis" that combines the results of 57 large prospective studies of all-cause mortality and BMI (Whitlock et al. 2009). Prospective studies provide the strongest research design to analyze this issue. The data in Figure 6.3 summarize the

112

FIGURE 6.3
Body Mass Index (BMI) and Mortality

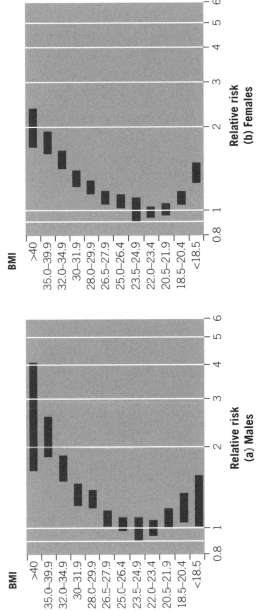

Source: Data from *The Lancet*, Vol. 373 [March 28, 2009], Prospective Studies Collaboration, "Body-mass index and cause-specific mortality in 900,000 adults: collaborative analyses of 57 prospective studies," pp. 1083–1096. Copyright © 2009 Elsevier. Data used with permission from Elsevier.

results from their meta-analysis (their Figure 2.1) that brings together the experiences of over 900,000 individuals.

For both men and women, the best survival rates appear in the groups with BMI of about 23 to 25. The relative risk climbs both for people with lower and higher weight than this "most-protective" BMI.[4] But (as the data in Figure 6.2 show), our problem in the United States is not an epidemic of underweight, but just the opposite—it's an epidemic of obesity. These data also show the higher risk that men face at any BMI. At the best BMI, men have a relative risk of 1.6 compared with the best-risk women. This partly comes from smoking histories, and partly from hormonal and other biological differences between men and women.

Obesity also causes numerous disorders that degrade the quality of life. Both obesity itself and its associated diseases reduce people's ability to do many of the enjoyable things in life. It increases the risk of hypertension, heart disease, numerous cancers, diabetes and its many associated diseases (vision problems, skin breakdown, further risk of heart disease), sleep apnea, abdominal hernias, gout, and varicose veins, just to hit the high points on the list. The risk of diabetes triples for people who are obese, and half of all hypertension patients are obese. Bringing body weight into normal ranges (BMI of

---

4. Relative risk shows the risk of death relative to the comparison group, so the best-BMI women have a relative risk of 1.0 and all others show the risk of death relative to that group.

about 23 to 25) could eliminate about 40 percent of all heart disease.

Obesity also makes it harder to do many of the simple things in life. Obese people can't easily fit into normal airline or movie theater seats. It's hard to find a wide selection of super-size clothing. It's harder to climb stairs, take a hike, play tennis, or do many other fun things in life. Obesity and exercise even affect sexual performance through a number of mechanisms (including diabetes and hormonal changes) to the extent that physically active middle-aged men have 70 percent less chance of later getting ED than do sedentary similarly aged men.

Quality of life (QOL, as self-reported in the Medical Expenditure Panel Survey done regularly in the US) declines markedly with smoking and obesity. These data show about a twenty percent loss in quality of life (at all ages) for obese smokers compared with non-obese non-smokers (Stewart, Cutler, and Rosen, 2009). Thus (for example) where 1 is perfect health and 0 is the worst possible health state imaginable, non-smoking non-obese persons of ages 45–54 reported an average QOL score of .84 and the comparable-aged smokers reported QOL scores of .74 (obese) and .69 (morbidly obese, BMI > 35).

Obesity also costs a lot of money. A recent analysis pegged the costs of obesity-related diseases at nearly $150 billion per year (Finkelstein et al. 2009). The average obese person uses about $1,500 per year more in medical services than a person of normal weight. That's about a 40 percent increase in medical spending compared with a non-obese person. About half of the extra cost is paid by taxpayers through public programs.

This is an issue everybody should care about, whether or not they are overweight. Our tax dollars are at issue through the funding of Medicare and Medicaid, and the costs of our private insurance go up in the same way because obese people pay the same premiums as non-obese people. Like smoking, obesity affects us all.

Alcohol

Alcohol is a perplexing drug. While many deaths, injuries, and illnesses come directly from excess alcohol consumption (liver disease, numerous cancers, vehicle crashes, interpersonal violence, etc.), substantial evidence also shows that moderate alcohol use—particularly wine and most particularly red wine high in tannins—actually protects humans against heart disease.

To understand the health effects, we need to bring two concepts into the picture. First, the real health problems come with heavy drinking and binge drinking.[5] Heavy drinking is known to increase the risk of various cancers, liver disease (particularly alcoholic cirrhosis),

---

5. Heavy drinking is commonly defined as more than twenty drinks per week. Binge drinking has a variety of definitions, the most common being five drinks (four for women) within a two-hour period.

and heart disease. Binge drinking affects vehicle crashes, interpersonal violence, and other conditions.

However, almost ironically, regular *moderate* alcohol use seems to have a series of health-protective aspects, particularly with regard to heart disease, more so when the alcohol of choice is wine, and especially so for some red wines with high levels of particularly beneficial complex chemicals.[6] A large study of Danish adults (Grønbaek et al. 2000) found that heavy drinkers of distilled spirits had about double the cancer risk of non-drinkers, but those who drank wine moderately (not heavy or binge) had a 20 percent lower all-cause mortality rate and almost cut the risk of heart disease in half (compared with non-drinkers).

Fighting the wrong drug war

Our official war on drugs focuses on various addictive substances such as marijuana, cocaine, heroin, and similar drugs. For a variety of historical reasons, these drugs became illegal early in the twentieth century.[7] However,

---

6. The key ingredient appears to be *procyanadin* (Corder 2007). For those who prefer to avoid alcohol, foods with high levels of procyanadin include chocolate, cranberry juice, pomegranates, and various apple species. It seems that an apple a day *does* keep the doctor away, at least for some apple species.

7. Both heroin and cocaine sales were legal until 1914, and they became controlled substances only in 1970. Cannabis (marijuana) became illegal in 1937. Bayer Pharmaceuticals actively sold heroin from 1898 until 1910 for pain control and coughs.

they account for less than 1 percent of all deaths in the United States. By contrast, tobacco causes 18 percent of the deaths in our country every year. Alcohol adds another 3.5 percent, for a total of 21.5 percent for these two legal drugs. This means that tobacco and alcohol account for thirty times as many deaths each year as do illicit drugs. Tobacco alone accounts for more than twenty-five times the number of deaths as do illicit drugs.

If we were to count obesity as an addictive problem (as some people do), we could add another 16.6 percent to the deaths associated with addictive behavior: tobacco, calories, alcohol, and illicit drugs. Together, they cause 39 percent of the nation's deaths. The conclusion leaps from the page: we're fighting the wrong drug war. The big health issue isn't illicit drugs, it's tobacco, obesity, and (in more complicated ways) alcohol.

The European paradox

Some people have asked me, "If smoking and obesity are the real issues, why don't the Europeans (and the Japanese, and so on) have health care costs higher than ours, since they smoke at much higher rates than we do?" Good question! I wish I had a perfect answer, but I only have several ideas to help think about the issue.

First, if they smoked less, the smoking/risk data almost guarantee that their health costs would fall. Second, we're just beginning to reap the benefits of the gradual decline in smoking rates in the United States.

118

Further, the Europeans mostly have implicit or explicit rationing mechanisms in their health care systems that put a lid on costs in a way that selectively saves costs due to smoking. Part of this comes from the observation that smokers die early in their lives, before developing other potentially expensive diseases (Manning, Keeler, Newhouse et al. 1989). But in most European societies, deaths that in the United States would involve expensive hospitalization, cancer treatment, and intensive care don't get treated the same way. For example, in the United States, half of all deaths involve intensive care, whereas in Great Britain, only one in ten deaths involve a stay in an intensive care unit (Wunsch, Linde-Zwerble, Harrison et al. 2009). ICU use for cancer is three to four times higher in the United States than in Britain, and eight times higher for strokes, two of the main "death certificate" causes of death for smokers.

The long-run fix

To solve this problem, we almost surely need a massive investment in public and private resources to find biologically based measures to help people alter their behavior, most notably tobacco use and overeating. Urging people to change their ways will not suffice. We have had some modest success in reducing smoking through public awareness, restrictive rules about smoking in public, higher taxes, and increased availability of pharmacological products (e.g., nicotine patches) that help reduce the craving while people withdraw from smoking.

We have had far less success in dealing with obesity. The epidemic proportions of increasing obesity attest to this problem. So also do the countless ads for weight loss programs, some based on caloric control, planned menus, diets high in carbohydrates, diets low in carbohydrates, low-fat diets, balanced diets, group support, and the like. Some products offered for sale hint at effective weight loss from various "natural" substances, usually with a warning such as "results not typical" next to the "before" and "after" photos.

Very few FDA-approved medications are available for weight loss. This highlights the problem: in order to claim that a drug helps people lose weight, the FDA has this nasty habit of requiring scientifically valid proof. Most weight-loss programs can't sustain the losses people achieve initially. Herbal and other remedies are not subject to FDA approval and hence claims made about these diet aids are not nearly as controlled as are those for prescription drugs.

The FDA has approved several weight loss drugs, including one prescription medication that affects the brain's hunger signals. The first over-the-counter (OTC) weight loss drug was approved in 2007; it works by blocking the body's ability to absorb fat. Therein lies the rub: what goes in must get burned or come out. Those who take this drug and eat fatty foods often have a *very* sudden reminder that they've recently eaten some fat.

For the dangerously obese (usually defined as those with BMI > 40), a relatively new approach called bariatric surgery shrinks or bypasses the stomach so that the person feels full after eating less. This works well for some people, but has potential side effects of acid reflux and (with overeating) nausea and vomiting.

There's an old joke in the economics profession: two economists are walking down the street, and one sees a $100 bill lying in the gutter. As he leans over to pick it up, the other admonishes him, "If it were a real $100 bill, somebody would have picked it up already." Diet aids are like that: if there were a diet aid that really worked and kept weight off forever, it would dominate the market. Instead, we see herbs and spices, various non-prescription drugs, acupressure and acupuncture, group therapy, individual counseling, exercise programs, meditation, many different surgical interventions, and numerous other approaches to reducing weight. Americans annually spend $33 billion on weight loss products and aids, about $150 per adult per year. Yet we still collectively gain weight at an astonishing rate.

Where's the beef?

Success in dealing with the adverse health consequences (death, illness, injury, pain, work loss, productivity loss)

121

and associated medical costs of these lifestyle choices will probably require a massive investment in basic research to better understand the causes, treatments, and prevention of key addictive and behavioral choices— tobacco and obesity most prominently, and alcohol abuse as well. It is just not happening right now.

We undertook just such a national endeavor beginning with President Johnson's war on heart disease, cancer, and stroke, and with massive increases in funding through the various National Institutes of Health to study the causes and cures of these diseases. These have paid great dividends in reductions of mortality and morbidity, as Chapter Three outlined.

The funding priorities of the NIH show just how far behind we are on the issues of tobacco, alcohol, and obesity. In slightly rounded numbers, the 2009 NIH budget provides $30 billion for all endeavors. Of this, $5 billion goes to the National Cancer Institute (NCI), $3 billion to the National Heart, Lung, and Blood Institute (NHLBI), and $1.6 billion to the National Institute of Neurological Disorders and Stroke (NINDS), adding up to almost a third of the NIH budget. These figures are byproducts of the 1960s war on heart disease, cancer, and stroke.

By contrast, NIH funding for the National Institute on Alcohol Abuse and Alcoholism rests at $0.4 billion. The National Institute on Drug Abuse received $1 billion in funding in 2009. We have no national institute to deal with tobacco addiction or obesity. While, to be sure, some of the NCI, NHLBI, and NINDS funds go toward prevention research, these agencies' research agendas are dominated by "cure" approaches.

I suggest that one of the best ways to reduce federal and private health care spending over the next fifty years would be a massive investment in federal research to find effective ways to eliminate tobacco use and excess caloric intake (obesity). This cannot succeed if done half-heartedly. That's what we have now.

In 2003 the NIH formed an Obesity Task Force that published a strategic plan to deal with obesity. It talks about cross-cutting research and emphasizes the need to deal with behavioral modification, pharmacological approaches, surgical approaches, etc. Astonishingly, the 114-page document contains only two examples of a dollar sign. One refers to the $117 billion in annual lost wages from the consequences of obesity. The other refers to the $33 billion spent annually by U.S. citizens on obesity and weight control products. Not a single word appears to suggest allocations of funds toward the question of obesity. Nobody is in charge. An old saying (in a particularly inept choice of metaphors in this case) goes, "If you assign two people to feed a dog, it will starve to death." That's where we are in the NIH with obesity.

NIH research directly focused on tobacco and nicotine use has a similarly dismal history. In 2000, one study looked at every grant issued by the NIH (across all institutes) to estimate the research funding directly focused on tobacco and nicotine use. The 1995 total (the most recent year of data) showed $95 million in dedicated research on this issue, less than one half of one percent of the NIH extramural budget.

Therein sits the stark contrast. We spend about a third of the NIH budget on trying to cure heart disease, cancer, and stroke. We spend less than half of 1 percent on prevention associated with tobacco use. Where things actually stand with respect to obesity research is unknown, but the fact that the strategic plan for dealing with obesity within the NIH utters not a single word about budgetary commitment speaks volumes.

CHAPTER 7

Why is Our K–12 Educational System a Public Health Menace?

As Chapter Six showed, long-term health outcomes for most individuals depend greatly on their lifestyle choices. Yes, good health care can often improve and sometimes cure the problems created by our lifestyle choices or our genes. But avoiding the problems in the first place solves many issues; we feel better and spend less on health care. That would be a win-win situation, for sure. Until genetic medicine comes of age, we can't do much about the mess our parents made of our genes, but we can do something about the lifestyle issues.

One of the best ways to improve the population's lifestyle is to improve our pre-college (K–12- educational system, which is widely understood to badly lag much of the developed world (NAS, 2007). Education is a wonderful preventive medicine. More highly educated people are healthier in many ways. The mechanisms by which this happens have not yet fully emerged, but several things seem clear now:

- Better educated people have higher incomes on average, hence they live in better situations, have better health insurance (to the extent that matters), and live in safer communities.

- Better education improves people's ability to cope with our very complicated health care and health insurance systems.

- Perhaps most important, highly educated people have better health habits. In particular, they smoke less, have less obesity, consume alcohol in healthier ways, and exercise more.

Let's review these health habits in more detail and then see if we can come to understand how better education improves health habits in particular.

Tobacco use falls rapidly as education increases. Using the most recently available data, for example, about 20 percent of the U.S. population smokes cigarettes. The education profile is remarkable, as Figure 7-1 shows.

The same education gradient appears even among health care workers. Those with the lowest educational requirement (licensed practical nurses, typically one year beyond high school) have a 27 percent smoking rate. Next come registered nurses (at least a two-year AA degree, often a four-year college degree), who have an 18 percent smoking rate. Physicians (college, medical

FIGURE 7.1
Current Smoking Rates by Education

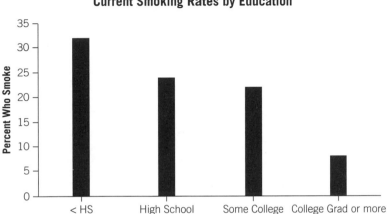

Data source: Health United States, 2009, US Department of Health and Human Services, National Center for Health Statistics, Hyattsville, MD, 2010, Table 60.

school, residency training) have only a 3 percent smoking rate.

We saw in Chapter Six that alcohol has complex effects on human health. Binge drinking (drinking with the goal of getting drunk) and heavy drinking (more than twenty drinks per week) are bad for your health, but moderate drinking (particularly wine) seems to protect one's health. Given that, let's look at drinking patterns by education.

In stark contrast with the patterns we see between education and smoking, here we see a strong link between final education level and alcohol use. The more education people have, the more they drink. Isn't this an

FIGURE 7.2
Education and Alcohol Use

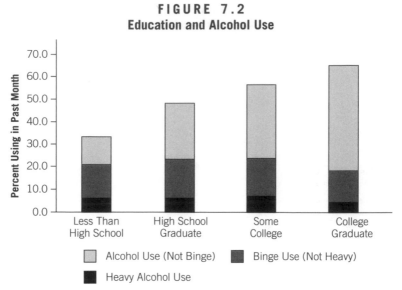

Data source: 2007 National Survey on Drug Use & Health, Table 2.45, Substance Abuse and Mental Health Services Administration.

anomaly in contrast to the tobacco story? Upon finer inspection, no. Moderate alcohol use, particularly avoiding binge drinking, has protective effects for health, most prominently for heart disease. Figure 7.2 shows a declining rate of heavy and binge drinking as education rises even though overall drinking rates climb with education.

The final link in the alcohol-education-health story comes from observing the beverages of choice by education. The more highly educated people become, the more likely they are to choose wine. So as education rises, the rate of drinking in moderation rises (protective in general) and the rate of drinking wine instead of other

128

FIGURE 7.3
Education and Obesity

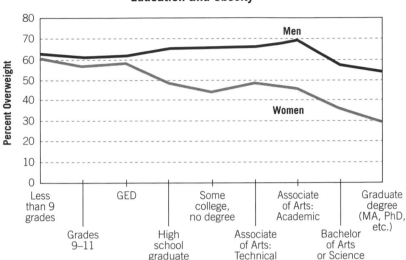

Data source: Percent of U.S. adults who were overweight (including obese) (BMI >= 25) and percent who were obese (BMI >= 30), by selected characteristics,1997. U.S. National Center for Health Statistics, 2002.

alcoholic beverages also rises. Combining these facts, we can see that alcohol fits the general pattern here—more education leads to behaviors that are health-enhancing.

Obesity is closely linked to education as well. Obesity rates (as measured by Body Mass Index) decline as educational attainment rises. The real protective effect seems to come only with college education for men, but begins at lower levels of education for women. Even at the highest levels of education, over half of the men in the United States are at least overweight, compared with about a third of women with college degrees or higher.

As an earlier chapter showed, the effects of excess weight are much larger for those with higher levels of BMI. Data from the most recent National Health Interview Survey show that the percentage of the population who are obese (BMI of 30 or higher) stays at about 30 percent for all groups with less than a college education, but falls to about 18 percent for those with college education or more.

Overall activity level affects weight, cardiac fitness, and other health outcomes. Inactivity is bad for you, more activity is better. Activity level closely relates to education, as Figure 7.4a shows.

Figure 7.4b shows the basic picture—higher education leads to more frequent vigorous *leisure* exercise (defined as at least ten minutes of vigorous leisure activity). The first observation is that very little of this actually transpires, possibly explaining the obesity levels in our society.

The picture, however, is more complicated than one might think at first glance. And it's quite different than what we see with smoking, in some important ways. Most obviously, people with more education are less likely to engage in manual labor, which often contains a hefty dose of what exercise gurus call a "vigorous workout." People who work in construction, day labor, and even apparently benign activities such as janitorial services and housecleaning all have relatively high rates of caloric burn during the day, and (more important for exercise physiology) often have at least one period of the day with an elevated heart rate—the key to good health

130

FIGURE 7.4a
Activity Level and Education

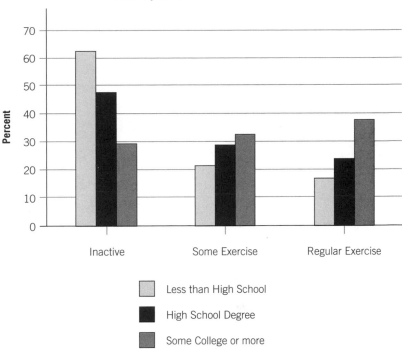

Source: Health, United States, 2008, Table 74

outcomes from exercise. So in some sense, lower-educated people are less likely to need to engage in leisure-time vigorous exercise to maintain their health.

The big surprise comes because (on average) the vigorous exercise "costs" people more when they have a higher education. This occurs because education raises the value of one's time, both within the market (higher wages and salary) and outside of the market (as people

FIGURE 7.4b
Education and Vigorous Exercise

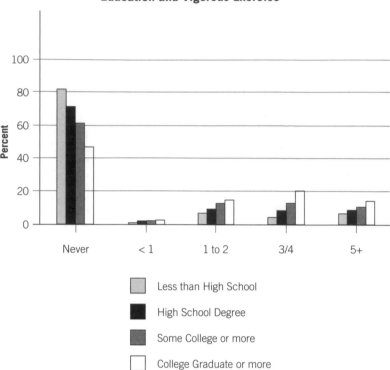

Source: CDC, 2008, Table 29

balance the value of their work and leisure hours). So to take an hour a day for jogging, cycling, or swimming truly is more costly for people with a higher value of time. This key point (Lakdawalla and Phillipson 2002) probably accounts for a significant amount of the increasing obesity we have seen recently. As time becomes more valuable (as it does with more and more education), peo-

132

ple find it more expensive to exercise for the purpose of shedding calories.

What creates the education/health link?

We don't know for sure if better education *causes* these outcomes or if some hidden trait (such as the way people value things "today" versus far in the future, called "global time preferences" by economists) leads to both the lifestyle choices and the education. Indeed, it may be that education alters people's time preferences.

The economics literature contains many analyses seeking to determine if more education indeed leads to better health, rather than just being observed together. This literature includes many natural experiments (mandatory increases in education through time, even twin-twin studies, which particularly attracted me since I have an identical twin brother). My reading of this extensive literature tells me that better education does indeed *cause* better health.

The link may come from a simple rational calculation involving the protection of an investment. If you have a car worth $10,000, you are less likely to buy a house with a garage to protect it from the elements than if you own a $50,000 car. The garage costs the same in either case, but it's worth more to protect the more expensive car. If you wear expensive Italian leather shoes, you are more likely to wear rubber boots in the winter to protect them from slush and salt (people living in the Sunbelt will have to excuse this analogy as irrelevant) than if you wear lower cost shoes. The same should happen with education—once people have invested in the quality of their brains, they should logically take better care of them, since a more highly educated brain is more valuable through the years.

The link may come from a more obvious source: people with better education may be able to assimilate information about health risks better than those with less education. We have several "natural experiments" that help shed light on these issues. The first came in 1964 when the U.S. Surgeon General issued a major report summarizing the available evidence that tobacco use created serious health problems.

The Surgeon General's 1964 report affected different parts of the population in very different ways. Literacy, reading habits, ability to understand presentations of scientific data, and a general belief in the scientific method probably all contributed to this process. We can see this process unfolding in post-1965 responses to the Surgeon General's report.

Figure 7.5 shows smoking participation rates by educational attainment for 1965 to 2005. In 1965, the lowest smoking rates occurred among college graduates, and the highest among those with some college education, with high school graduates and those with less than high school in between. These patterns in 1965 show the combined effects of education, income, peer group behavior, and other factors.

FIGURE 7.5
Smoking Changes by Educational Level

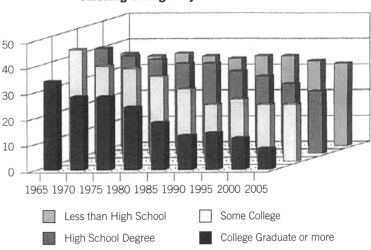

Data source: Health United States, 2009, US Department of Health and Human Services, National Center for Health Statistics, Hyattsville, MD, 2010, Table 61.

The most remarkable feature of this graph is how differently smoking rates changed over time by educational attainment. Here we see a perfect match between education and response to the information. Those with less than a high school education (the back row in the graph) maintained almost the same smoking rate from 1965 forward for the next four decades. Those with a high school diploma (the next row forward in the graph) started out a bit higher, but cut smoking rates considerably. Those with some college education cut even more, and those with a college degree both started out with the lowest rate and had the greatest reduction in smoking rates.

Thus it seems that adding new information to the market has little effect on the decisions of individuals with low levels of education, but a much more powerful effect on those with the highest level. If the information helps people understand the risks of some behavior (such as smoking cigarettes), it seems that those with more education can systematically evaluate that information and use it to alter their behavior at a much greater rate than those with less education. The (smoothed) annual response rate for college graduates is over ten times larger (3.5 percent annual decline) than for those with less than a high school education (0.3 percent annual decline).

A separate "natural experiment" is now under way in China. Because of dramatic investments in educational systems by the Chinese government beginning about a quarter-century ago, educational levels in China have steadily increased. For example, between 1985 and 2005, the proportion of Chinese with at least some post-secondary education increased from under 3 percent to more than 20 percent. More than 70 percent of Chinese children now enroll in high school, up from under 40 percent in 1985.[1] What has happened to health habits during the same time?

The results—by now no surprise—show smoking and heavy drinking rates have fallen dramatically among Chinese adults. The proportion of those over age fifteen who smoke has dropped from 33 percent in 1993 to 26 percent in 2003, an annual rate of decline of 2.4 percent.

---

1. These data come from the World Bank's EdStats resources.

The proportion of Chinese adults who drank heavily also fell considerably during the same ten-year period (China Daily 2004). Beginning in January 2010, seven cities in China will ban smoking in public places to prevent health problems from secondhand smoke (China Daily, 2010). These data again show how increased education brings with it a reduction in smoking rates.

Conclusion

We can see a strong link between education and health-promoting or health-protective behaviors. Does education cause this or do we just see a correlation with something else (say, time preference)? Several things reviewed earlier in this chapter suggest causation, notably the patterns of smoking cessation by education following the 1964 Surgeon General's report and falling tobacco use rates as education increases in China, where the increase is driven by policy, not individual choice. Numerous formal studies in the economics literature support this conclusion.

The strong links, even if only partly caused by education, make it imperative that we strengthen our abysmal K–12 education system. How to do this? I refer readers to the many excellent publications by the Koret Task Force on K–12 Education of the Hoover Institution for the answer to this puzzle; it's beyond the scope of this modest work on health and health care.

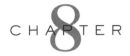

C H A P T E R

Where Does the Congress Miss Opportunities and Hit Potholes?

We have left undone those things we ought to have done,
And we have done those things we ought not to have done,
and there is no health in us.

(Prayer of Confession)

Let's use the ideas in this book to look at the health care reform legislation under development in Congress at the final stages of writing this book. We can first observe that what is widely described as "health care reform" is really "health insurance reform" and not much more. To be sure, it's the right place to start, but many important tasks remain undone.

First, the proposed legislation systematically increases the amount of insurance coverage, not only by extending coverage to most, but not all, of the uninsured (undocumented aliens have fallen through the cracks, for example) but also by mandating increases in minimum coverage. This last step in particular goes in the wrong direction. Our nation already has too much insurance in many ways.

The 2009 Senate Health Committee bill set minimum coverage at 76 percent of the total allowed costs of a particular benefit, while the Senate Finance Committee chose 65 percent. The House bill split the difference at 70 percent. None of the proposals discusses high-deductible plans as a solution, although they all include catastrophic cap protection (a good thing) at various levels. The mandated coverage percentages will very likely increase demand and health care costs for at least some citizens, not to mention the increased use of care for those who become newly insured through the reforms.

Various forms of the proposals also embed employer premium payments into the law, the highest requirement appearing in the 2009 House bill, with a mandate that employers pay for at least 72.5 percent of employees' premiums. The Senate Health Committee opted for a 60 percent requirement. The Senate Finance Committee included no such requirement. These requirements obviously institutionalize the system of employer-paid premiums (coupled with the tax subsidy therein) that has led to so many distortions and excessive insurance through the years, as well as creating other economic disturbances in the labor market.

On the "left undone" side, Senate proposals would tax "Cadillac" insurance plans with an excise-tax arrangement (35 percent excise tax on plans costing more than $8,000 for individuals, $21,000 for families). But none of the proposals deals with the exemption of employer premiums from the income tax base. These proposals have drawn the wrath of both the insurance industry (the tax is to be paid by the insurers, who presumably will pass along the cost to their customers) and labor unions, which have long fought for very generous health benefits for their members.

Other areas of true reform did not really enter the debates. Nothing deals with the widespread variations in medical care use, an area of potentially enormous gains in reducing medical costs without adverse health risks. Nothing deals seriously with health habits, either by funding priorities for government research or by creating incentives for individuals through taxes or linkages of health insurance costs to lifestyle choices. Private insurance has successfully done this for decades with respect to smoking for life insurance, homeowners insurance, and disability insurance. Nothing but political will stands in the way of doing similar things for health insurance with respect to smoking, obesity, and alcohol use.

Nor has anybody tackled the issues of information and education about the effects of obesity. The cumulative effects of numerous legal changes, research findings, educational campaigns, and, finally, public sentiment have greatly changed the landscape of tobacco consumption, almost all for the better in terms of both health outcomes and health care costs. This should give us hope that a similar campaign—necessarily one probably spanning decades—can help resolve the growing epidemic of obesity and its associated health problems and medical care costs.

The process of introducing new technologies into the health care system has essentially remained outside the sphere of discussion, although most health economists (myself included) believe that technological change accounts for much of the "real" (inflation-adjusted) growth in medical care spending.

Beginning with the congressional mandate in 1964 that Medicare cover procedures that are "necessary and reasonable," the discussions about covering new drugs, devices, and procedures have been almost devoid of cost considerations, quite in contrast to the British National Health Service use of cost-effectiveness analysis in coverage decisions. Recent news events suggest that our political system will have great difficulty in dealing with these concepts, even though cost control sits at the heart of much of the economic and political debates about the merits of various reform proposals.[1] For now, it seems

---

1. In November 2009, the U.S. Preventive Services Task Force cut back on the age group for which it recommended mammography screening for breast cancer, shifting the recommended starting date from forty to fifty. Judging from the political response, one might think it was recommending infanticide. A former head of Health and Human Services urged that the recommendations be ignored. Senate hearings began almost immediately, and the White House made a special statement to assure people that government programs would continue to cover mammography for women under age fifty.

difficult, if not impossible, to bring cost considerations into coverage decisions in our health care system.

Thus the reform legislation, however it comes out, represents the beginning, not the end, of a journey. Hopefully, this book will help readers better assess future proposals and think more clearly about the issues involved in reforming our health care financing system and the entire health care system more broadly.

For those of you who have had your appetite whetted for a deeper understanding of health care and reform, I recommend another book produced by the Hoover Institution's Working Group on Health Care Policy: *Health Reform Without Side Effects: Making Markets Work for Individual Health Insurance*, by Mark V. Pauly (Hoover Press, 2010). I also modestly commend to you my textbook, *Health Economics*, fourth edition, wherein many of the ideas in this book are explored in greater depth.

REFERENCES

Anderson, G. "Chronic Conditions: Making the Case for Chronic Care," Johns Hopkins University Partnership for Solutions, September 2004.

China Daily, "Cities Set to Order Ban on Smoking," January 10, 2010, http://www.chinadaily.com.cn/china/2010-01/18/content_9333453.htm.

China Daily, "China Smoking Dramatically Dropped: Survey," December 2, 2004, www.chinadaily.com.cn/english/doc/2004-12/02/content_396825.htm.

Congressional Budget Office, "Effective Marginal Tax Rates on Labor Income," Washington, DC: US Government Printing Office, November 2005.

Corder, R. *The Red Wine Diet: Drink Wine Every Day and Live a Long and Healthy Life*, New York: Penguin Press, 2007.

Dartmouth Atlas of Health Care, 2009, online: www.dartmouthatlas.org.

DiMasi, J.A., R.W. Hansen., and H.G. Grabowski. "The Price of Innovation: New Estimates of Drug Development Costs," *Journal of Health Economics*, March 2003; 22(2):151–85.

DiMasi, J.A., R.W. Hansen, and H.G. Grabowski. "Extraordinary Claims Require Extraordinary Evidence," *Journal of Health Economics*, September 2005; 24:1034–1044.

Finkelstein, E.A., J.G. Trogdon, J.W. Cohen, and W. Dietz. "Annual Medical Spending Attributable To Obesity: Payer- and Service-Specific Estimates," *Health Affairs* 2009; 28(5):w822–w831.

Fisher, E.S., D.E. Wennberg, T.A. Stukel et al. "The Implications of Regional Variations in Medicare Spending, Part 2: Health Outcomes and Satisfaction with Care," *Annals of Internal Medicine* 2003; 138:288–298.

Gaynor, M., and P. Gertler. "Moral Hazard in Risk Spreading and Partnerships," *RAND Journal of Economics*, winter 1995; 26(4):591–613.

Giertz, S.H. "How Does the Elasticity of Taxable Income Revenues Affect Revenues and Economic Efficiency and What Implications Does This Have for Tax Policy Moving Forward?" in *Tax Policy Lessons from the 2000s*, A.D. Viard, ed., Washington, DC: American Enterprise Institute, 2009.

Goonzer, M. *The $800 Million Pill: The Truth Behind the Cost of New Drugs*, Berkeley, CA: University of California Press, 2004.

Grønbaek, M., U. Becker, D. Johansen et al. "Type of Alcohol Consumed and Mortality from All Causes, Coronary Heart Disease, and Cancer," *Annals of Internal Medicine*, September 2000; 133(6):411–419.

Gruber, J. and M. Owings. "Physician Financial Incentives and the Diffusion of Cesarean Section Delivery," *RAND Journal of Economics*, spring 1996; 27(1):99–123

Hall, R.E. and C.I. Jones. "The Value of Life and the Rise in Health Spending," *Quarterly Journal of Economics* 2007, 122(1):39–72.

Helms, R.B. "Tax Policy and the History of the Health Insurance Industry," in H.J. Aaron and L.E. Berman (eds), *Using Taxes to Reform Health Insurance*, Washington, DC: Brookings Institution, 2008.

Hickson, G.B., W.A. Altemeier and J.M. Perrin. "Physician Reimbursement by Salary or Fee-for-Service: Effect on Physician Practice Behavior in a Randomized Prospective Study," *Pediatrics* 1987; 80(3):344–350.

Hillman, B.J., C.A. Joseph, M.R. Mabry et al. "Frequency and Cost of Diagnostic Imaging in Office Practice: A Comparison of Self-Referring and Radiologist-Referring Physicians," *New England Journal of Medicine* 1990; 323:1604–1608.

Kaiser Family Foundation, http://www.statehealthfacts.org/profileglance.jsp?rgn = 1.

Lackdawalla, D. and D. Phillipson. "The Growth of Obesity and Technological Change: A Theoretical and Empirical Examination," Boston: National Bureau of Economics Research Working Paper No. 8946, April 2002.

Lee, S.H., G. Russo, et al. "The Effect of Mandatory Employer-Sponsored Health Insurance on the Use of Part-Time versus Full-Time Workers: The Case of Hawaii," 2009, http://www.allacademic.com/meta/p90630_index.html.

Light, D.W., and R.N. Warburton, "Extraordinary Claims Require Extraordinary Evidence," *Journal of Health Economics* September 2005; 24(5):1030–3.

Madrian, B.C. "Employment-Based Health Insurance and Job Mobility: Is There Evidence of Job-Lock?" *Quarterly Journal of Economics* 1994; 109:27–54.

Manning, W.G., E.B. Keeler, J.P. Newhouse et al. "The Taxes of Sin: Do Smokers and Drinkers Pay Their Way?" *Journal of the American Medical Association* 1989; 261(11):1604–1609.

McGinnis, J.M. and W.H. Foege. "The Actual Causes of Death in the United States," *Journal of the American Medical Association* 1993; 270(18):2207–2212.

Mitchell, J.M. and E. Scott. "Physician Ownership of Physical Therapy Services: Effects on Charges, Utilization, Profits, and Service Characteristics," *Journal of the American Medical Association* 1992, 268(15):2055–2059.

Mokdad, A.H., J.S. Marks, D.F. Stroup et al. "Actual Causes of Death in the United States, 2000," *Journal of the American Medical Association* 2004; 291(10):1238–1245.

National Academy of Science (NAS), *Rising Above the Gathering Storm: Energizing and Employing America for a Brighter Economic Future*, Washington, D.C.: National Academies Press, 2007.

Newhouse, J.P. et al. *Free for All? Lessons from the RAND Health Insurance Experiment*, Cambridge, MA: Harvard University Press, 1993.

Nguyen, N.X. and F.W. Derrick. "Physician Behavioral Response to a Medicare Price Reduction," *Health Services Research* August 1997; 32(3):283–298.

Pauly, M.V. *Health Reform Without Side Effects: Making Markets Work for Individual Health Insurance*, Hoover Press, 2010.

Phelps, C.E. "Diffusion of Information in Medical Care," *Journal of Economic Perspectives*, 6(3), summer 1992:23–42

Phelps, C.E., *Health Economics*, Boston: Addison Wesley, 2010.

Qato, D.M., C.G. Alexander, R.M. Conti, et al. "Use of Prescription and Over-the-counter Medications and Dietary Supplements among Older Adults in the United States," *Journal of the American Medical Association* 2008; 300(24):2867–2878.

Skinner, J. and J.E. Wennberg. "Exceptionalism Or Extravagance? What's Different About Health Care in South Florida," *Health Affairs* August 13, 2003.

Stewart, S.T., D.M. Cutler, and A.B. Rosen. "Forecasting the Effects of Obesity and Smoking on U.S. Life Expectancy," *New England Journal of Medicine* 2009: 361(23):2252–2260.

Whitlock, G., S. Lewington, P. Sherliker, et al. "Body-mass Index and Cause-specific Mortality in 900,000 Adults: Collaborative Analyses of 57 Prospective Studies," Prospective Studies Collaboration, *Lancet* 2009, 373:1083–1096.

Wunsch, H., W.T. Linde-Zwirble, D.A. Harrison et al. "Use of Intensive Care Services During Terminal Hospitalizations in England and the United States," *Critical Care Medicine* 2009; 180: 875–880

Yip, W. "Physician Responses to Medical Fee Reductions: Changes in the Volume and Intensity of Supply Coronary Artery Bypass Graft (CABG) Surgeries in Medicare and the Private Sector," *Journal of Health Economics* 1998; 17(4):675–700.

ABOUT THE AUTHOR

CHARLES E. PHELPS received his BA in Mathematics from Pomona College in 1965, an MBA (Hospital Administration) in 1968 and PhD (Business Economics) in 1973 from the University of Chicago.

Phelps began his research career at the RAND Corporation in 1971. During his time there, he helped found the RAND Health Insurance Study and served as Director of RAND's Program on Regulatory Policies and Institutions.

In 1984, Phelps moved to the University of Rochester, with appointments in the Departments of Economics and Political Science. From 1984–1989, he served as Director of the Public Policy Analysis Program. In 1989, Professor Phelps became chair of the Department of Community and Preventive Medicine in the School of Medicine and Dentistry of the University of Rochester.

In 1994, Professor Phelps was appointed as Provost (Chief Academic Officer) of the University of Rochester, a position he held until August, 2007. At that time, he was named University Professor and Provost Emeritus, positions he now holds.

In 1991, Professor Phelps was elected to the Institute of Medicine of the National Academies of Science, and also as Fellow of the National Bureau of Economic Research.

Professor Phelps has served on the Board of Trustees of the Council of Library and Information Resources (1998–2006, Chair 2004–2006) and the Center for Research Libraries (2004–2010). He also currently serves on the Board of Directors of VirtualScopics, Inc. He also serves as consultant to Gilead Sciences and CardioDX, and is a member of the Working Group on Health Care Policy at the Hoover Institution at Stanford University.

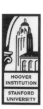

WORKING GROUP ON
HEALTH CARE POLICY

The WORKING GROUP ON HEALTH CARE POLICY will aim to devise public policies that enable more Americans to get better value for their health care dollar and foster appropriate innovation that extends and improves life. Key principles that guide policy formation include the central role of individual choice and competitive markets in financing and delivering health services, individual responsibility for health behaviors and decisions, and appropriate guidelines for government intervention in health care markets.

The core membership of this working group includes Scott W. Atlas, John F. Cogan, R. Glenn Hubbard, Daniel P. Kessler, Mark V. Pauly, and Charles E. Phelps.

INDEX

health care workers, 126–27
health insurance
    after World War II, 73–74
    Cadillac plans, 85, 140–41
    capitation, 38–39
    carve-outs, 42, 101–2
    case payment, 39–42
    case review, 43–44
    catastrophic risk protection, 35
    coverage decisions, 69–70, 142
    deductibles, 34–37, 65–66
    effect of, 36f
    employer-provided, 18, 19, 47,
        63, 73–82, 75n2, 75n3, 79n7,
        81n8, 82, 84–85, 84n11,
        140–41
    exclusions to, 79–80
    fraud, 33
    gatekeeper plans, 47
    hassles of, 46–47
    high-deductible, 65–66
    incentives by, 98, 141
    insurance markets, 82–84
    lack of, 19
    lump sum payments, 38
    no deductible, 66
    over-insured, 82
    patient incentives, 64–66, 103
    pay for performance, 44–46
    payout system, 16–17
    portability of, 80
    premiums, 83
    provider incentives, 66–67
    RAND HIE study of, 34–37,
        36f
    reform of, 82, 85, 139–41
    risk with, 31–33, 37, 102
    sources of, 17–19
    stop loss, 34
    under-insured, 82–83
    universal employer coverage,
        78–79

Health Insurance Portability and
    Accountability Act (HIPAA), 80
health maintenance organizations
    (HMOs), 38
    with Medicare, 46n6, 64n6
    in RAND HIE, 39
Health Savings Account, 37n2
heart attacks, ix
heart disease, 51
    NIH prioritization of, 51n1
    from obesity, 114–15
    pharmaceutical drugs for, 52
    wine and, 116, 117, 127–28
heart surgery, 52
heavy drinking, 116–17, 116n5
    in China, 136
heroin, 117n7
HIPAA. *See* Health Insurance
    Portability and Accountability
    Act
HMOs. *See* health maintenance
    organizations
Hollywood, 110
hospice care, 41
hospitals
    decrease in, 51
    DRGs in, 39–42
    length of stay in, 20–21, 39,
        40–41
    market share of, 20–21
    Medicare payments to, 21
    not-for-profit, 22
    operating cost of, 19, 19n7
    profit, 22
Hungary, health care spending
    infant mortality, 7f
    life expectancy, 6f, 8f
    national income and, 3f
hypertension, 56t, 114

Iceland, health care spending
    infant mortality, 7f

157